Praise for *Awakening Somatic Intell*

"All of us find ourselves confronted with the tension between having a body and being some-body. We have to meet the challenge of integrating these two ways of relating to our body. Dr. Kaparo's book can help us accomplish this integration and reap the fruits of mind-body wholeness. For this help she deserves sincere gratitude."
   —DAVID STEINDL-RAST, Benedictine monk, cofounder of gratefulness.org, and author of *Gratefulness, the Heart of Prayer: An Approach to Life in Fullness*

"If all of Dr. Kaparo's research and experience led to nothing more than expansion of your spine, the implications for your health would be enormous. Chiropractors should take huge notice. Her work, developed from her own personal healing journey, helps you experience the oneness of your body and spirit. Awakening to this essential truth can lead to a personal transformation in healing and conscious awareness."
   —ROBERT JAY ROWEN, MD, editor in chief, *Second Opinion Newsletter*

"Dr. Kaparo's passion for awakening and how that relates to the human nervous system has revealed many practical applications for all those who are exploring this new horizon. The inclusion of sensations and somatic intelligence assists in allowing the conversation between our older brain and the cortex to come into alignment, which allows for the embodiment of awakening. Her work and expression of what she has discovered in her journey resonates with the latest research that is helping so many. May her contribution benefit all beings."
   —ISAAC SHAPIRO, author of *Outbreak of Peace, It Happens by Itself,* and *Burning Questions*

"This book is a precious gift to those who are open to healing and transformation. It is also the fruition of many years of work filled with Dr.

Kaparo's dedication and heart. I pray that it reaches and helps many people."

    —ANAM THUBTEN RIMPOCHE, author of *No Self No Problem*

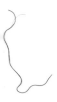

"Dr. Kaparo is a true original, and a genius at getting results. *Awakening Somatic Intelligence* offers the surprising keys to transforming your physical structure from the inside out. You will never experience your body the same way again because of the deep context Kaparo offers. This is a book that is on the leading edge of psychology, neurology, biology, and mindfulness."

    —STEVE BHAERMAN, coauthor (with Bruce Lipton) of
        Spontaneous Evolution: Our Positive Future and a Way to Get
        There from Here

"Dr. Kaparo outlines an exquisite feedback system to enhance and accelerate the benefits of mindfulness-based practices, laced with the strength of her compassion and dedication to her compelling work. This comprehensive book is a culmination of her discoveries and insights; she shows us how to love those who are suffering—right into their own healing."

    —TRUDY GOODMAN, founding teacher of InsightLA and
        contributing author of *Compassion and Wisdom in Psychotherapy:*
        Deepening Mindfulness in Clinical Practice, Clinical Handbook of
        Mindfulness, and *Mindfulness and Psychotherapy*

"Though Dr. Kaparo's work is still new to me, I almost immediately recognized her work as a missing link between the physical and spiritual. She has been the only one who has guided me to an understanding of how these two aspects, physical and spiritual, interpenetrate and are one and the same. She then gives a map to explore this as a real practical experience, not just philosophy. Because the path to her understanding was entirely experiential, she has been outside any spiritual system, which showed me how the spiritual is inherent in nature, not something born of Eastern or Western spiritual or religious traditions.

"This knowledge almost immediately switched my inquiry away from looking for the 'spiritual' or being on a path, to having an appreciation and direct experience of the vast beauty that I am composed of, and the incredible intelligence that is the foundation of my being. I have been able to relax and trust the process of awakening for the first time, not as something to figure out, but as something to rest in and savor. This understanding has allowed my potential and talents to be actualized much quicker, and has accelerated my authentic creative process."

—DEMIAN MCKINLEY, somatic therapist and internationally renowned yoga teacher

"Research in the areas of neurological plasticity, interpersonal neurobiology, and sensorimotor/somatic treatment of traumatic states has only recently—often with the advent of cutting-edge instrumentation—validated and replicated the concepts and methods presented here, discovered by Dr. Kaparo over thirty years ago. Kaparo deserves recognition as a pioneer; she is the only person of whom I am personally aware who has formed her ideas through both her personally developed rehabilitation and subsequently applied and validated clinical experience in transformational healing. Her system is unique."

—STAN FRIEDMAN, PhD, clinical psychologist in private practice, Los Angeles, California

"In her excellent book, Risa Kaparo shares with readers her process of 'learning to navigate the ocean of life' through a series of contemplative exercises that allow the reader's mind-body experience to release and awaken to the freedom that is our true nature. This is one of the most comprehensive presentations available of learning how to be in the active experience of moment-to-moment 'presencing,' getting in touch with the subtleties of one's own physical, non-dual integration with life itself. I highly recommend this wise and nuanced book that needs to be read a number of times to glean the fullness of its wide spectrum of wisdom teachings. This is a great addition to one's personal library of spiritual guidance."

    —RABBI DAVID A. COOPER, author of *God is a Verb: Kabbalah and the Practice of Mystical Judaism*

"This book represents a breakthrough in healing the mind/body split. It offers an artful, exquisitely subtle and integrated way of navigating the interior of the bodymind that is naturally good medicine as well as a means to greater awakening."

    —DANA ULLMAN, regular writer for *The Huffington Post* and author of *The Homeopathic Revolution: Why Famous People and Cultural Heroes Choose Homeopathy*

Awakening
Somatic
Intelligence

The Art and Practice
of Embodied Mindfulness

Transform Pain, Stress, Trauma, and Aging

Risa F. Kaparo, PhD

Forewords by Rick Hanson, PhD,
and James Oschman, PhD

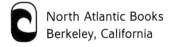

North Atlantic Books
Berkeley, California

Published by
North Atlantic Books
P.O. Box 12327
Berkeley, California 94712

Cover photo © iStockphoto.com/Photokdk
Cover and book design by Suzanne Albertson

Printed in the United States of America

Awakening Somatic Intelligence: The Art and Practice of Embodied Mindfulness is sponsored by the Society for the Study of Native Arts and Sciences, a nonprofit educational corporation whose goals are to develop an educational and cross-cultural perspective linking various scientific, social, and artistic fields; to nurture a holistic view of arts, sciences, humanities, and healing; and to publish and distribute literature on the relationship of mind, body, and nature.

North Atlantic Books' publications are available through most bookstores. For further information, visit our website at www.northatlanticbooks.com or call 800-733-3000.

PLEASE NOTE: The creators and publishers of this book disclaim any liabilities for loss in connection with following any of the practices, exercises, and advice contained herein. To reduce the chance of injury or any other harm, the reader should consult a professional before undertaking this or any other movement, meditative arts, health, or exercise program. The instructions and advice printed in this book are not in any way intended as a substitute for medical, mental, or emotional counseling with a licensed physician or healthcare provider.

Somatic Meditations, Somatic Intelligence, and *Somatic Learning* are service marks owned by Risa Kaparo, PhD. For all rights and permissions, please inquire at www.awakeningsomaticintelligence.com.

Library of Congress Cataloging-in-Publication Data

Kaparo, Risa.
Awakening Somatic Intelligence: the art and practice of embodied mindfulness /
Risa Kaparo.
     p.; cm.
     Summary: "A valuable resource for readers seeking to improve their health and well-being, *Awakening Somatic Intelligence* introduces Somatic Learning, an innovative healing approach rooted in body awareness that incorporates the latest research in psychology, neuroplasticity, and mindfulness"—Provided by publisher.
     ISBN 978-1-58394-417-2 (pbk.)
I. Title. [DNLM: 1. Mind-Body Therapies—methods. 2. Awareness. 3. Meditation. 4. Psychophysiologic Disorders—therapy. WB 880]
     615.5—dc23   2011038944

1 2 3 4 5 6 7 8 9 SHERIDAN 16 15 14 13 12
Printed on recycled paper

For Deanna,
and the generations to come
and
in memory of
Vanda Scaravelli

I dedicate this book to the awakening of all beings.
And to all the teachers who have come before.

Acknowledgments

I bow to my beloved friend and mentor, Brother David Steindl-Rast, who taught me about gratefulness and leisure. He said, "Leisure is the expression of detachment with regard to time," and "leisure … is not the privilege of those who can afford to take time, it is the virtue of those who give to everything they do the time it deserves to take."

When I first met Brother David, a Benedictine and Buddhist monk, he asked me about my practice. I told him that though I had begun a very serious Buddhist practice in 1969, it changed in 1979, after I had the opportunity to participate in some dialogues with Jiddu Krishnamurti. Since then I have been traveling a pathless path … learning to, as Krishnamurti often said (using the words of Buddha), "Be a light unto oneself." Though I have been touched profoundly by wisdom teachers from many traditions, I do not follow any religion. Instead, my life has evolved into a daily, serious commitment to the art and practice of awakening, in which all the activities of life, all my relations, and indeed all of nature serve as portals to deepen presencing spaciousness. Brother David said it is not that I do not have a tradition, it's that I come from a perennial tradition: the tradition of universal mystics.

That said, the passionate inquiry that has sustained my attention for more than forty years was informed by the many disciplines I pursued, and the many wonderful mentors that the "river of service" carried my way. I bow with gratitude in this section to my own lineage and the teachers who have most personally and profoundly touched my life. For those interested in the many friends and mentors who have influenced the development of this work, I refer you to a second list of acknowledgments at the end of this book.

Bowing in all directions:

I bow in honor to my family, for the precious gift of sharing this life together. And to all my ancestors (Eastern European Jews) who lived through extremity and discovered *"What can you give that can never be taken?"*[1] I reclaim their courage and call upon their blessing in making this offering to you, for what we presence now is the only reason we ever exist. I bow to my daughter, Deanna. The intensity of love I feel for her continues to inspire me to transcend all barriers.

I bow in honor of my beloved teachers. In passing on their legacy to you, I call upon the invisible umbilicus of the great lineages they embodied to provide refuge and nourishment for you. First, to the Buddha, the Dharma, and the Sangha, a deep bow. To all my Buddhist teachers, spanning forty years of practice, especially to Thich Nhat Hanh, Sakyong Mipham, Lama Tsewong Sitar, Anam Thubten, Trudie Goodman, Daniel Brown, and Tenzin Palmo.

To Jiddu Krishnamurti, who transformed my practice through the gift of choiceless awareness. To his dear friend, the theoretical physicist David Bohm, who provided me with a scientific foundation for my healing and transformational work, and a deeper understanding of our system of thought. I have had the grace of sharing many inquiries with him and Krishnamurti, as well as with the other pioneers who have driven the art of dialogue into modern practice—Carl Rogers, Patrick DeMari, and Bill Isaacs—while I developed one of the disciplines of *Somatic Learning* as a form of social meditation, *Covenants of Co-Presence: A Yoga of Dialogue.*

Krishnamurti also introduced me to another dear friend who became my teacher of the heart, Vanda Scaravelli. I bow to her with the warmest affection. She guided me in practicing yoga that transformed my relationship to gravity and time. I could sum up her teaching with one koan: Infinite time, no ambition. No ambition, infinite time.

Though she challenged me with very strenuous practices from the beginning, she could hardly bear to see me effort. A breakthrough occurred when I stopped *trying to do* what she asked of me and started sensing as she sensed, receiving the support of gravity and the ground, sensing the wave of interpenetrating movements, and presencing spaciousness with each breath. I am most grateful for the extraordinary opportunity to live with and practice alongside her several hours each day on and off across a quarter of a century. Had I been limited to the hourly lessons she gave other students I don't know if I ever could have learned so much from her. A bow to her teachers, BKS Iyengar and TKV Desikachar, and their teacher Sri T. Krishnamacharya, who brought forth the teachings from their devotion to practice.

Moving back from Europe, I took another year of sabbatical from teaching to deepen my inquiry while living with two remarkable people: Emilie Conrad Da'oud and Gary David, PhD. Their friendship has been a blessing beyond words. I bow to Emilie, the visionary behind Continuum Dance Meditation. Emilie and I shared a passion for embodying spaciousness, and our exploration of intrinsic movement often carried us into uncharted seas. I cherish both her sisterhood and her work. Gary, a brilliant and creative teacher of Epistemics—a methodology for developing awareness of meaning-making—opened my eyes to the process of abstraction. I bow to him and his teacher, Samuel Bois, and his teacher in turn, Alfred Korzybski, founder of General Semantics. My dialogues with Gary, spanning some thirty years now, have also deepened my understanding of Affect and Script Theory. I bow as well to his teachers, Donald Nathanson and Silvan Tomkins.

I bow to the next generation:
To the therapists, educators, students, and clients who I have had the honor of guiding and who have been my greatest teachers throughout the years. I want to especially thank the students and practitioners of Somatic Learning who supported my writing of this book and production of videos, contributed their own writing, and participated in photo sessions. They include Shosanah, Neil, Tore, Chanterel, Beorn Chantera, Lisa Chipkin, Tatiana and Humberto De Blanco, Reka Foss, Carrie, Scott, Tyler, Gage and Kolea Rautman, Sophie and John Alexander, Nancy Margulies, Martin Mazzanti,

Toni Mazzanti, Ron Harwin, DC, Jarvin Heiman, MD, Mark Wilson, OMD, Andrea Fuchilieri, Kat Zandvakili, Larry, Anna Marie, Margaret and Katherine Boucher, DJ Colbert, David Andrighetto, Katherine Elijah, Katrama Brooks, Sharee Anderson, Shakira, Mark and Pua Freeman, Steve, DJ and Angelie Star, Tim Star, Steve and Trudy Bhaerman, Shakti Gawain, Robert Rowen, MD, Joan Levy, Joan and Andrew Thompson, Ursula Lamberson, Elaine Valios, Gitta and Kane Mirkus, Alain and Jody Herriott, Patrick Deluz, Peter Clarke, Jeff Groethe, Leslie Deluz, Frieda Elliot, Paula Jeane, Pam and Clarke Bell, Stan Nielson, Julie Ireland, Sally Mabelle, Ron Moshontz, Chad Bennett, Ellen Wolfe, Carol Yamasaki, Aki Creelman, Joelle Yzquierdo, Adrienne Mohr, Teresa Lumiere, Lynn Dhority, and Shavan Bill Peay.

A bow to my friends:
To my dear friends Kay Snow Davis and Robbie Engleman, who passed on during the writing of this book … with whom I share such sweet sisterhood.

To Lisa Alpine, a co-conspirator with whom I shared my first writing office and began this manuscript some thirty years ago. To Gail Shafarman, PhD, the brilliant psychologist, poet, and writer with whom I have had the privilege of sharing an office over the last twenty years and on whose wise counsel I have grown to depend. To my dear friend, David Surrenda, PhD, with whom I began to write one version of the manuscript and with whom I would enjoy any opportunity to co-create. To Donna Genuth, a student of mine, who asked if she could sit with me when I wrote. Her lovely presence allowed me to write to a real person with whom I felt a deep heart connection rather than a hypothetical audience.

To my devoted protégé Steve Star, who offered to continue to sit with me in Donna's place when she left the island, and continued to work with me on retreat for weeks at a time for several years. The field of his unwavering interest inspired my writing with the intimacy of two friends walking through a garden together, lavishing on each other all the joys expressed in nature and companionship. His attention allowed me to meander non-linearly, following the inspiration of what emerged, without fear of losing the thread of meaning. I can hardly express the extent of my gratefulness and joy in passing this transmission on to him, practicing alongside one another the way I practiced with Vanda.

To all those who generously offered support and editorial advice along the way: Dana Ullman, Shakti Gawain, Christina Crawford, Ellen Wolfe, Steve Bhaerman, Sherrin Bennett, Larry and Anna-Marie Boucher, Bill Unger, Stan Friedman, PhD, Stuart Bell, Joyce Jenkins, Sarah Ackerman, Josh Hecht, Peter Howard, Carla King, and especially David A. Lawrence, PhD, for his brilliant editing support. To Michael Malter and Peter Beren for their legal and publishing advice.

And to Sergio Baroni, my gratefulness for the sincerity of his deep interest and wild enthusiasm, which helped me place the finishing touches on the manuscript with fresh eyes. His loving devotion and wise reflections drew forth onto these pages the voice of poet he celebrates in me.

A bow with the deepest gratitude to Charles Davis for his photography and art videography. And for their artistic contributions: Brian Zeiglar in photography; Maurice Wren, Danny Hashimoto, and Jeremy Sutton in painting and photography; Jeffrey Townscend, videography; Ralph Adamson, paintings; Richard Greninger, videography; and the drawings of Nancy Margulies.

To Andrew Alvarez, my multi-talented angel, whose skills and calm, generous presence have assisted me in almost every aspect of completing this work.

To my editors Jessica Sevey and Kathy Glass, designer Suzanne Albertson, and all the wonderful folks at North Atlantic Books, for their kind attention.

To Rick Hanson, PhD, and James Oschman, PhD, for contributing their heartfelt forewords.

To Suzanna Gratz, my dear friend and agent from Inspiring Promotions, who has continued to empower and inspire me in bringing this work out into the world.

Last but not least, I bow to you, dear reader. I can hardly express the overwhelming sense of gratitude I feel for all the extraordinary teachers I've been blessed to have. But you do not have to travel to the four corners of the Earth in order to understand and engage somatic intelligence. Having devoted my life to this learning, it gives me great pleasure to bring the harvest of these practices and great wisdom traditions to you in the form of this book.

> Oh, the comfort, the inexpressible comfort of feeling safe with a person, having neither to weigh thought nor measure words, but pouring them all right out, just as they are, chaff and grain together, certain that a faithful hand will take and sift them, keep what is worth keeping, and with a breath of kindness, blow the rest away.
> —*Dinah Maria Craik, from the poem, "Friendship"*

Contents

    Contents

Foreword

By Rick Hanson, PhD, author of *Buddha's Brain: The Practical Neuroscience of Happiness, Love, and Wisdom*

In Western cultures, there's been a historical tendency to approach the human body in two contradictory ways: to exploit it as a source of pleasure, yet also to label it as sinful and categorically distinct from the "loftier" mind.

Happily, in the last few decades a variety of intellectual, psychological, and spiritual efforts have emerged to bridge these two approaches in order to provide a more integrated engagement with the body. For example, philosophers and neuroscientists alike have moved beyond Descartes's mind-body dualism, psychologists have produced studies in the emerging field of "embodied cognition," and therapists have created powerful body/mind treatments for trauma and other issues.

Dr. Kaparo's book builds on and adds to these developments, grounded as it is in both the latest findings of brain science and the ancient wisdom of the perennial traditions. A master clinician, she has a rare gift for bringing sophisticated ideas down to earth and weaving them together with simple and practical things people can do to make their body wiser—and thus their lives better. She has a genius—a word I don't use lightly—for both the body and its language.

An explosion of research over the past decade has revealed the power of the mind to change the structure of the brain. For example, studies have shown that the mindful attention Dr. Kaparo offers to readers can literally thicken the cortex in two key regions, building millions of new synapses in the anterior (frontal) cingulate cortex—which increases the control of attention and the integration of thinking and feeling—and in the insula, which increases both self-awareness and empathy for the feelings of others. Additionally, the deepening warmheartedness and intimacy one experiences with oneself and others through her practices are associated with increased flows of oxytocin, a neurotransmitter and hormone that supports love and bonding.

In her book, Risa Kaparo offers reverence for the natural wisdom of the body, the nurturing guidance of a great therapist, and a detailed operating manual for healing pain and awakening embodied joy. I have benefited personally from her work, and commend it highly to your attention.

Foreword

By James L. Oschman, PhD, author of *Energy Medicine:*
The Scientific Basis

> Movement and art inspire each other. The creative process of
> inhabiting one's art, one's movement, and one's life is the same.
> —*Barbara Mindell*

At an early age, I became fascinated with the explorers who were the first
to go where no one had gone before. My first visit to a library led me to
Half Mile Down by William Beebe. I was enthralled with his descriptions
of luminescent deep-sea creatures never before seen or even suspected to
exist. I felt like I was with him in his bathysphere, exploring mysterious new kinds of life, and sharing in his rapture and amazement with
the astonishing creatures inhabiting and illuminating the deep dark sea.
What an adventure!

A comparable excitement will grip all who survey the depths of
life revealed by another of the truly great explorers of our times, Risa
Kaparo. Here the watery depths of self and relationships are plumbed
by an adventurer of great courage and wisdom—a journey comparable
in surprises and excitement to those experienced by other fearless souls
who have, down through the ages, exposed the hidden places on and
within our planet and within ourselves. Following Dr. Kaparo on her

journey of discovery does not require a bathysphere or a rocket ship or a microscope—it only requires a vehicle we all possess, a human body, with all of its mysteries that few have explored as deeply and thoroughly and lovingly as Dr. Kaparo has. It is thrilling that she has taken the step of sharing her journey with all of us in this brilliantly written book. It is obvious that her courage in exposing the depths of the bodymind comes from an abiding love and affection for all who would follow the journey she has opened for us.

It is an honor that some of the explorations I have made with my wife, Nora, illuminate parts of Dr. Kaparo's remarkable journey. The scientific research she quotes represents a synthesis of insights from many different disciplines. Our key discovery is the interconnectedness of *the living matrix*—the molecular fabric that extends throughout our bodies and that is the core and essence of what we refer to as *holism*. For our bodies mirror the continuous and interconnected framework of nature at all levels of scale, from subatomic particles to distant galaxies.

The living matrix concept arose from the study of the microscopic anatomy and interconnectedness of our cells and tissues, combined with observations and insights of the therapists who interact with the human body through touch, energy, and movement. The living matrix records all our traumas, both large and small, the stresses and strains of life, injuries, diseases, emotional attitudes, choices, and habits. Operating silently in the background of our normal neurological awareness, the "matrix consciousness" provides the foundation for experiencing our inner and outer selves. The wounds we experience accumulate and compromise our creativity, joy, and longevity. Somatic Learning is Dr. Kaparo's way of bringing awareness to our hidden reservoirs of compromised structure and movement, enabling us to turn back the clock to the remarkable, integral functioning we were born with. The self-renewal process does not involve fixing things so much as it involves restoring our innate perfection and infinite potentials. There is a synergy to this process, meaning that as one piece of our being is restored to full vitality, the others tend to fall into alignment. The emerging field of epigenetics teaches us that the results of Somatic Learning percolate via the living matrix into our DNA, switching particular genes on and off. All who practice the methodology developed by Dr. Kaparo, including practitioners of any form of therapy, will benefit from the practical wisdom contained in this book.

The living matrix is just a concept, useful to some but unknown to many. Dr. Kaparo has animated the matrix—brought it into life and motion. Her tools are simultaneously creative, intuitive, and poetic—an expanding dynamic synthesis. In her work, she operates at the delicate and mysterious interface between the known and the unknown. It takes courage and deep trust of the powers of intuition to walk this edge without falling, a process Dr. Kaparo refers to as *presencing,* a process all who read this book can learn and master. All who embark on such a journey will enjoy their own direct experience of astounding insights and outcomes.

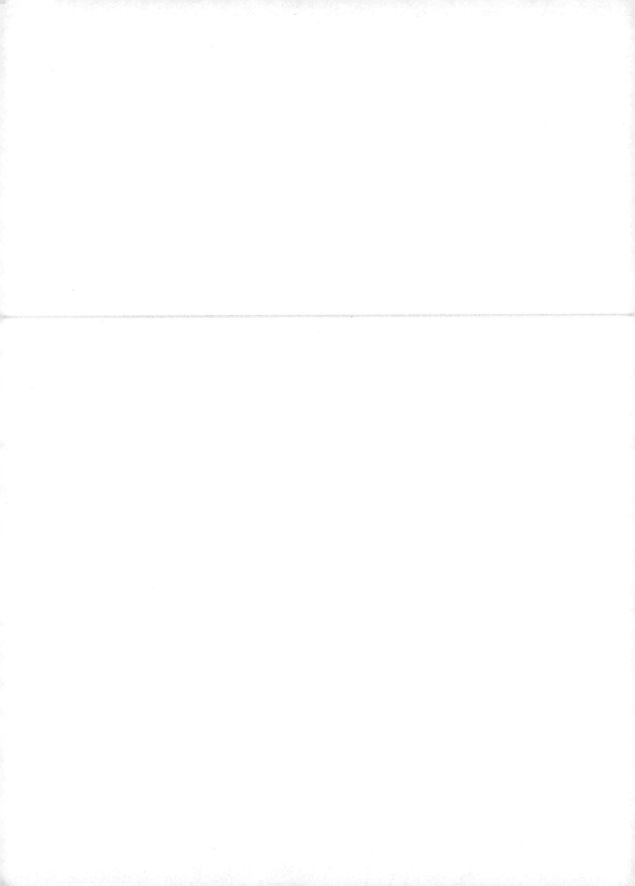

Introduction
Insights from the Ancients

For many years, I looked out upon the magnificent Pacific from my home on the island of Kaua'i, and felt inspired by the ancient Polynesians who migrated eighteen hundred years ago from the Marquesas to the Hawaiian Islands.[1] Imagine you are one of them, kneeling in a dugout canoe, without the aid of navigational equipment. Your ancestors found a slipstream that carried them the distance across the Pacific to these tiny islands surrounded by more than two thousand miles of sea in all directions. Since your dugout canoe holds so few provisions, the accuracy of your navigation is the difference between life and death for your *ohana*—all your relations—on board. How would you navigate?

The "wayfinders" had many tools for navigation: reading the stars, wind, smells, taste, sensing the temperature variations of the ocean currents. But changing weather patterns could render any or all of these unreliable. Somehow, the ancient navigators learned to sense the streaming of this deep current in the vessel of their bodies, by resting their testicles—the most sensitive part of their body—on the base of the canoe. They did not accomplish the migration by paddling hard against the current, but by relying on their own astonishingly sophisticated information sensing, processing, and course-correcting organisms.

You can learn to engage the same innate wisdom of embodied mindfulness to skillfully navigate into a new life now, just as the ancients did. Engaging somatic intelligence will serve you in all aspects of living—from giving birth to dying—transforming pain, stress, trauma, and aging. It can break the endless cycle of addiction to substances, food, work, and dysfunctional relationships. Somatic intelligence engenders ever-greater freedom and aliveness while enhancing your happiness, compassion, and capacity to love.

This flies in the face of our conditioning to ignore the signals from our bodies as we focus on achieving a goal. When they lost the slipstream, the ancient navigators sensed the change in pressure through their own bodies, allowing them to deftly correct course. So too, when you listen to the signals from the vessel of your body, you learn to sense your loss of connection to the slipstream of joy and interest that had been sustaining you. When you recognize yourself tensing toward an accomplishment, there is no secondary act of will necessary for change. When you see that the tension actually takes you in the opposite direction of the movement of your deepest longing, you stop pressurizing yourself, and disenthrall from the illusion that straining will lead to a better moment. When you are naturally loving what you love, there is no arrival, and nowhere to get to. Whatever you are engaged in serves as a perfect portal to awakening in this very moment, just as it is.

Extending the Legacy

This book is a deeply personal invitation, from my heart to yours, to explore Somatic Learning, the art and practice of awakening somatic intelligence. It's an invitation to receive your birthright—the natural wisdom of embodied mindfulness—as the compass from which to navigate your life any time/anywhere you are, from how you think and feel, see and speak, read and write, eat, heal, drive, rise in the morning and fall asleep at night, how you relate to all beings, to our beautiful planet. Every place you find yourself can serve as the perfect learning environment to awaken to the infinite spaciousness that you are.

Like the ancients, you can learn to navigate the ocean of life from the vessel of your body, as you recapitulate this journey of the soul in your own life today. Conscious evolution necessitates sustaining connection with the infinite. Aligning your innate somatic intelligence (sensing) with the growing edge of what is possible (the slipstream) opens you to what yearns to be born within the movement of your becoming. We not only learn to receive the unbounded spaciousness, but our gratefulness finds expression in being fruitful ... as we give birth to ourselves anew.

Turning Urgency to Gravity

This book offers a practice that brings immediacy to presencing the unbounded source of all existence. In *Somatic Learning* I use the term *presencing* as a verb to imply the embodying of spaciousness with awakened *Somatic Intelligence*. "Extending presence" refers to the process of living into the unknown, relaxed and curious, without efforting to grasp anything—aware of what happens in the bodymind as you ease the struggle to "wrap your mind around something." When we can be present or mindful as we live into the unknown, the infinite reveals itself to us so that we come to know it intimately.

The practice takes up the "urgency" one feels in stress, pain, or trauma—which is what most often motivates people to begin the practice. However, through the practice you learn to meet the challenge without reacting to it. You learn to "turn urgency into gravity" by awakening somatic intelligence, so that you can respond in creative, compassionate, and empowered participation. Since the only thing we have is now and now and now, all possibility of transformative learning and change (healing and realizing our wholeness) can only occur in the present. Nothing changes when we live in the meanwhile, waiting in hope for a better future.

Begin Beautifully, Begin Now

The practice begins with how you read and make meaning. This is an invitation, not a recipe book. As you read this, I encourage you to let the words enter into your experience as a lake receives raindrops. Don't distance yourself by analyzing what you read. Instead, feel the meaning rippling through you, settling into the depths of your intelligence so that you enter into a dialogue with the book rather than taking what is offered on authority.

As my beloved teacher Krishnamurti often related, dialogue can feel like two friends walking through a garden—feeling the firmness of the ground supporting our verticality as it rises through our feet, the radiance of the sun warming our skin, smelling the fragrance of flowering herbs carried on the breeze, hearing the tone and rhythm of our voices expressing meaning. This book arises out of a daily "dialogue with oneself" and with others that began some forty years ago, riding the waves of my joy and interest.

I will write to you the way I speak, and sometimes you will find ellipses … and dashes—leaving space for our breath to enliven, pause, suspend. You may find unexpected punctuation, indentations, and italics to highlight a shift in voice or mind perspective. And lines that do not follow the subject/predicate assumptions of grammar to form complete sentences or perhaps they run on, the meaning lapping gently over itself as it ripples outward, enfolding into your whole sense of significance and unfolding as new insight.

You may find unusual words that I will define for you (you can always refer to the glossary) or ordinary words not associated with their common, diluted usage but reclaimed to express the insights to which their etymological roots originally referred. These words may surprise you. Though familiar, they no longer fit neatly into the known. I know that my writing "style" tends to start with an insight expressed "all at once" and then to slowly unravel its meaning. So if you don't understand something you read initially, I invite you to ride the waves of your curiosity despite the uncertainty.

Hawaiians have twenty-eight words for moon; and an indigenous cir-cumpolar group, the European Sami People, have hundreds of words for snow[2] that support them in navigating their environment. By using language to refer to more specific, differentiated meanings, we can chart new territory together, navigating aspects of experience that have previously been uncharted. Words may serve as poetic referents, inviting you to leap from the known magically, through a rabbit hole, where you enter a new dimension—a wonderland—or alternate reality that parallels our consensual realm. Here you can leave behind the reductionism, determinism, and mechanistic thinking of our common-sense reality. You needn't get caught up trying to figure out what I mean, or comparing it to your past knowledge and experience. Let it re-member or "whole" you at a new depth of meaning, like a cloud can point you to sense the vastness of the sky.

How to Use This Book

As you may have intuited by now, this is not another health-and-fitness book. This book offers a lifetime of exploration into the extraordinary capacity for embodying mindfulness, as well as insight into transcending what limits us.

Part I, "Somatic Intelligence Is Your Birthright," introduces *Somatic Learning* conceptually. It presents new theoretical models and leading-edge research from emerging sciences. It includes an exploration of healing practices and many stories to empower you to employ creative ways of participating with the immediate real-life challenges you face.

In Chapter 4, we enter the metaphoric world of fairytale. This chapter explores how "the embrace" reveals our inherent beauty and renews us—symbolized by the transformation from old hag into beautiful young maiden. The story brings to life what happens when we lovingly embrace "what is"—we dispel the curse of fragmentation (or the belief that we are somehow separate from all that is). This chapter also distinguishes between achieving the temporary relief of "state-specific affects" and the process of integration into a self-sustaining, self-renewing order.

Part II, "Reorganizing Your Structure, Reorganizing Your Life," begins with breathing because it is at the heart of all the *Somatic Meditations*. *Somatic Learning* is an awareness practice that utilizes many different *Somatic Meditations*. The breath is the primary movement we return to when we notice that we're lost.

In the bedtime practices, both at night and upon arising, you can set an intention for your sleep or day that places "a stake in the ground." You will polarize the field around the energetic "ground" or intention that you set. Rather than chasing down each thing you have to get done throughout the day, your clear intention becomes the magnetic pole around which all action, activities, and relationships come into coherence. The Bedtime Practices chapter begins with an exploration of the sympathetic and parasympathetic branches of the autonomic nervous system and how you can simply and powerfully enhance your quality of life and well-being.

The morning practice is especially beneficial because you have rested and fasted through the night, and the mind is so quiet. The down time has rendered you more open to the restructuring at a much deeper level.

Starting your day with *Somatic Meditations* will empower you to enter the day non-reactively. From this state of alignment you will find creative ways to participate, proactively, in whatever challenges arise. I encourage you to notice this difference. When you develop a taste for it, you will become unwilling to settle for less. You will stop settling for a life of playing catch-up, reacting to external circumstances in an attempt to survive. Also, if you do not find time in the beginning of the day to set your day, to take ownership of it, it is more than likely that the day will get out of control. Thus, you will be less able to find time in the later part of the day, or you will be too spent and lack the necessary attention for practicing later.

This is not to say that if you miss your morning practice there is no point in beginning later—you can begin at any time. Each time you discover that you have lost yourself is the perfect opportunity to find yourself again and bring about a more coherent functioning, where the surface and the depths of your experiencing are congruent. When the surface of life—your thoughts, your behavior, how you function in the world—is congruent with the depths of your somatic intelligence, you will care for yourself and others joyously and live with ease.

Part III, "The Art and Practice of Somatic Learning: Anytime Anywhere Practices," offers *Somatic Meditations* you can practice with flexibility (i.e., anytime, anywhere)—so that you can learn to sustain the inquiry throughout the day. These practices also start very simply—though they have the potential of becoming infinitely subtle and profound. As you begin to practice, you will discover which somatic meditations best serve you at any given moment. You needn't have a long, drawn-out practice to gain benefit. Even one breath with awareness can relax your tension, or enhance your enjoyment and renew you when you feel depleted.

For example, in Chapter 12, "changing planes" is the generic term we use for movement from one position to another (for example, sitting to standing). The typical way people change planes comes from an adversarial relationship to gravity, much like handling a sack of potatoes, with lots of lugging, hoisting, leveraging, etc. Worse than all the "efforting," most of the body weight ends up precariously perched over some unsuspecting joint like a knee. When this house of cards tumbles, the over-weighted joint pays the price. Rather than being a "danger zone," changing planes can become an "awareness zone" where it is possible to safely and gracefully flow from one position in space to another, integrating a new paradigm—an alliance with gravity—into our structure and functioning.

Part IV, "Deepening Your Practice," offers insight into ways of enhancing one's practice through self-facilitation. With touch, you can provide more specific feedback to sense where and how you can release yourself.

Once you learn how to self-facilitate with your touch, not only can you amplify your own feedback anytime for yourself, you also learn how to touch someone else in a way that enables them to extend their presence. Eventually you will learn to transfer the sensation to different parts of your structure using your awareness alone, without needing the touch. There are places where it is impossible for you to touch yourself. However, as you tune into what it feels like to be touched and learn to move from that touch, you can create an invisible partner that provides this quality of touch for you.

I recommend that the first time you use this book, you do the practices in the order that they appear. We will develop the differentiations gradually, using each practice for refinement. As you continue following the guided Somatic Meditations, though the instructions remain the same your inner conscious awareness will become more differentiated, transforming your practice. Like all nature, "the body" is not a fixed entity; it will respond according to how you probe. Each day that you practice you will invent and discover a new body in relation to your state of consciousness.

Even with very limited free time, you can still enjoy these practices. Most can be done at any time, indoors, outdoors, at home, while out and about, or at the workplace. Starting the day with these practices takes advantage of the quiet with which you awaken.

The present book offers stages of differentiation. First, a more basic practice, then I add greater complexity and subtlety that continually deepen the practice so it can open infinitely. I invite you to self-regulate, taking up new differentiations and variations in a way that does not overwhelm you, while not allowing your practice to plateau. With this approach, you never repeat the same practice twice.

This book was designed to deepen your practice as you progress, so it will benefit you to work through it in a sequential way the first time. However, it was also designed to be used in a non-sequential way, to support you in referencing different sections according to your individual needs and interests. In the beginning, all the instruction will keep the conscious mind very busy. After you learn some of the Somatic Meditations "by heart" you can continue the process of extending your presence beyond the known to reinvent/discover yourself anew in each moment.

I encourage you to read through the practices first, drawing resources for yourself from all the supporting diagrams, photos, and references. You can also play the Somatic Meditations on audio and video formats available from www.awakeningsomaticintelligence.com, so you don't have to read the instructions while engaged in the actual practice.

You can see this book as a tree, the conceptual thread forming its trunk and providing a structure for the meaning to unfold in a more theoretical form. The conductive parables speak to us aesthetically, nourishing our deep feeling sense with their richness. These two, like sap and heartwood, must grow together to form a stable structure.

Branches extend from this trunk into various fields, each holding the potential of nourishing us in a different way. They carry the leaves of research and scientific theory, and evocative material such as poetry and art, as well as the stories of transformative learning and change experienced by people who have engaged in the practice of Somatic Learning.

Just reading, like looking into a canopy of leaves, will provide a perspective that will begin lighting up your participation differently. However, the best way to use this book is to ground the new learning in your own experience. The Somatic Meditations will serve as roots,

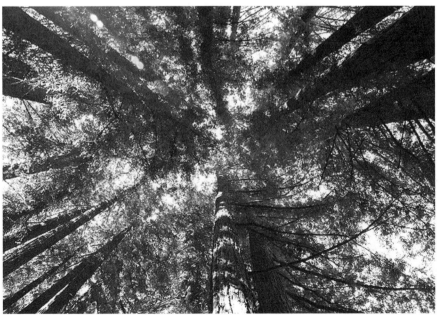

A different perspective

awakening a direct and immediate connection to your innate somatic intelligence. While practicing these meditations, you can extend into a greater dimensional awareness from the inside out as you read, rather than merely taking in the material inferentially. Let your silent-level experience serve as an ambient background to hold the different threads of meaning as a whole, providing an aesthetic reference for the art and practice of presencing.

This book is an invitation to live life to the fullest by awakening somatic intelligence. Enjoy the journey!

A sizeable body of research exploring the nature of consciousness, carried on for more than thirty years in prestigious scientific institutions around the world, shows that thoughts are capable of affecting everything from the simplest machines to the most complex living beings. This evidence suggest that human thoughts and intentions are an actual physical "something" with the astonishing power to change our world. Every thought we have is a tangible energy with the power to transform. A thought is not only a thing; a thought is a thing that influences other things.

This central idea, that consciousness affects matter, lies at the very heart of an irreconcilable difference between the worldview offered by classical physics—the science of the big, visible world—and that of quantum physics: the science of the world's most diminutive components. That difference concerns the very nature of matter and the ways it can be influenced to change.

—Lynne McTaggart, from *The Intention Experiment: Using Your Thoughts to Change Your Life and the World*

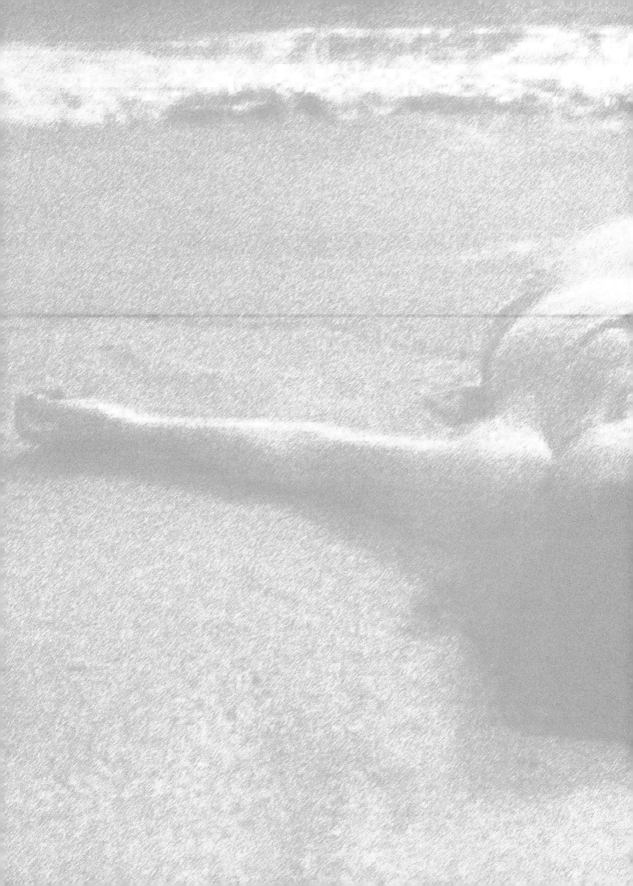

PART I

Somatic Intelligence
Is Your Birthright

Subatomic particles, and all matter made therefrom, including our cells, tissues, and bodies, are in fact patterns of activity rather than things.

—*Fritjof Capra*

How will you hold the rare and perilous given you?
Dawn begins in the bones
  —*Risa Kaparo*

CHAPTER 1

Dawn Begins in the Bones

This book is for people who seek ever-greater freedom and aliveness—people who will not settle for less than living the most creative, empowered, passionate, and compassionate lives possible. This book is written for you.

Paradoxically, you may have picked up this book because you are experiencing limitation—stress, pain, dis-ease, injury, and trauma, whether physical or psychological. Indeed, the pain of this limitation may be the very thing that impels your search for aliveness. Yet in time, you may come to see these challenges as a blessing: they bear the gift of necessity, elevating your search with a sense of urgency.

For more than thirty years, I have taught Somatic Learning, a practice for transformative learning, healing, and change through awakening somatic intelligence. In my experience, people often initially arrive at my door not because they are consciously aware of wanting to live a deeply sensed, awakened life—but because they are in pain.

Their conditions range widely. They may have an injury, structural problems, or a chronic illness. They may be grieving from a loss, suffering with depression, or wanting to feel a greater connection within themselves and the world. They may sense the possibility of a way of maturing gracefully rather than having degeneration and limitation characterize their aging. While some are interested in spiritual development and personal growth, that is not what usually compels them to come—at least not initially. What they want is to be free of pain.

Regardless of your motivation in coming to this book, what you will find in Somatic Learning is the transformative power of awareness: the power to release tension and struggle—to heal and renew—and to savor your experience in a way that enhances the grace, beauty, and enjoyment of life. Developing your somatic intelligence will enable you to heal, and to awaken ever-greater freedom and aliveness. As this innate intelligence takes hold, it will deepen your capacity to feel, and to sense yourself as fluidly embodied and connected—to the Earth and to the Infinite.

Your body is a supremely responsive and alive feedback system. When you begin to encounter it as an immediate presencing, rather than as an "object," your body opens up its song to you, and you become not only the music but also the instrument and the player.

> Movement is the song of the body. Yes, the body has its own song from which the movement of the body arises spontaneously. In other words, the liberation of the upper part of the body … produced by the acceptance of gravity in the lower part of the body … is the origin of lightness, and dancing is its expression. The song, if you care to listen, is beauty. We could say that is it part of nature. We sing when we are happy, and the body goes with it like waves in the sea.
> —*Vanda Scaravelli*[2]

The word "somatic" comes from the Greek root *soma,* for "body." The conventional use of the word "body" in English implies an "object" observed from the outside. It is a "third-person" image of ourselves at a distance. That's why I use the term "soma" to refer to how we sense the unfolding of life from within. And I use the term "somatic" to imply a first-person, here-now, all-at-once, embodied intelligence—how we sense, feel, and know ourselves on a process level—from the inside out. This is what we are in our fullness at "no distance" in contrast to a "third-person" image of ourselves at a distance. Confusing the map (image level) with the territory (process level) represents one of the fundamental sources of incoherence in our prevailing system of thought.[3,4]

Why is this gift of embodiment so important? Because we learn through feedback. We need this feedback to sense, evaluate, and respond intelligently. The feedback we receive through being born into a human body on this Earth provides us with the perfect learning environment to unhook from our misidentification with "object" reality and awaken to the infinite consciousness that we are. After all, we could not learn to swim on dry land. We need the resistance of water in order to sense our movement. And we need Earth's field of gravity in order to sense the support coming from the ground. Your somatic intelligence provides you with feedback from the most finely tuned feedback system ever imagined—feedback that is in real time and immediately apprehensible. In the words of Buddha, this is "knowing the body from the body," one of the four foundations of mindfulness.

If we are aware in the moment when we come to the intersection of two freeways, we can make the smallest adjustment to navigate the road while driving to stay on course. At the junction of I-80 and I-580, a simple lane change modifies my route. However, if I am not awake at that critical juncture, an hour later I will either be in Sacramento or San Francisco. The longer I travel along a route, the harder it is to self-correct. This is why Somatic Learning proves to be so valuable. It utilizes real-time feedback to support us in making the tiny shifts in awareness that alter the course of our lives, the state of our health and happiness both physically and emotionally.

Without developing our somatic intelligence as a guidance system, we may not realize the course we are on until we reach a destination we did not intend. At times, as with degenerative aging or injury, it may even prove to be a destination from which we cannot return. Obviously, it would behoove us to awaken the natural biofeedback guidance system that is our birthright before we wear out a hip joint or worse. Even when we are dealing with extremity, the self-health[5] practices of Somatic Learning can still prove miraculous, as the stories students share of their own experiences will reveal.

> Ring the bells that still can ring
> Forget your perfect offering
> There is a crack in everything
> That's how the light gets in
> That's how the light gets in
> —*Leonard Cohen*

My Healing Journey: From Crippling Pain to Ever-Greater Freedom and Aliveness

To introduce Somatic Learning and the power of Somatic Intelligence, I would like to share the story of my own journey—the healing that originally set me on this path.

Somatic Learning is not something I learned from a book or a teacher. I learned it from within my own body and consciousness, just as I will assist you in doing in this book. The willingness to pay deep attention to the inner wisdom and movement of your body is a fully sufficient teacher to move you into a state of utter wholeness and aliveness.

Like many things that eventually turn out to be wondrous discoveries, this journey was initially impelled by pain. My life changed radically when I "hit a wall" as a young woman. As an artist at the time, I had received a government commission to build a fiber-art playground on a Navajo reservation. We had to ground our structures in rock—shale, we'd been told, a fine-grained sedimentary rock, easy to drill. But as it turned out, it wasn't shale at all, but solid rock. With my hundred pounds of weight, I felt like a flag flying off the jackhammers, and my IUD (internal uterine contraceptive device) cut into my uterine wall. As I didn't want to disappoint the children with whom I lived on the reservation or my six apprentices, I worked throughout the ordeal until I finished the playground. But by that time, I could hardly move anymore, due to the intensity of the pain.

The injury led to an infection, and—with a pregnancy and loss of pregnancy—I developed pelvic adhesions (scar tissue in and between my organs) that would pull and tear with the slightest motion, leading to more internal bleeding and scar tissue. Walking was almost unbearable. I became bedridden and lived in constant pain.

The doctors insisted on a radical hysterectomy, since they were certain that the damage would make it impossible for me to ever have children. They warned me that because of the adhesions, they wouldn't know the impact until they opened me up. I was told that even after surgery it was very probable that I would continue to bleed internally and remain in pain.

Between the pain and the pain medication—which was taking me out of myself, distancing me from my body—I could hardly think straight. I had to find a way back to myself through the "underwater" effect that the medication was producing. I knew that the choices I needed to make would have enormous personal consequences. I forestalled the surgery, hoping to find a way to get off the pain medication or at least lower it enough just to think straight. I didn't know what to do. I was very young and desperate enough to try anything that might relieve my pain and avoid the radical surgery.

Led by the Blind

What I did to try to control the pain came from insights I had gained while teaching painting and sculpture to blind students a few years earlier. Most of my students had been blind from birth, and few had visual

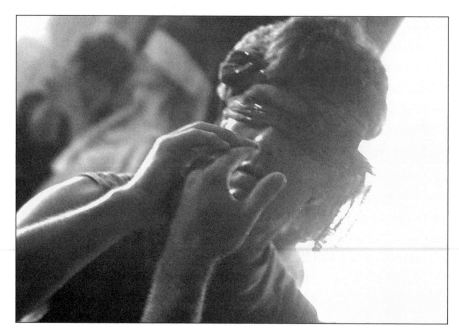

A workshop participant blindfolded for a Somatic Meditation

memories through which they could relate to the world—or to what I was attempting to teach them in class. After all, how does an individual who has never had sight experience his "arm"? I needed to find out how I could serve these students in my class.

I began by blindfolding myself to better understand their experience and discover ways to teach them. As I entered this world of not seeing, I started to understand that the search for how my blind students "saw" was not easy. It soon became apparent that I related to the world primarily through visual perception. At first, as I sat in the darkness, only memories and images projected themselves in my mind. I knew myself—my body—in memory, as if I were an image in the mirror. Finally, I had a breakthrough when I began to sense through my own actual bodily system (as opposed to my mental image of myself). As I began to experience myself outside the visual field of perception, I discovered that my whole being responded. For instance, if I sensed my arm, it was no longer the

Somatic Intelligence Is Your Birthright

arm as "object"—what I knew from my memory and imagination. It was a real-time sensing of movement within movements.

One day during that period, I woke with searing pain in my head. I was not sure where it came from. Despite the pain, however, I continued with my daily experiment of blindfolding myself. Soon I could sense movement—a throbbing. As I sensed into it, the throbbing began to change shape, elongate, become undulating pulsations. As these shapes changed, the intensity fluctuated and eventually diminished of its own, like a wave rippling outward. Gradually, the pain was no longer exploding through my head. Instead it became sharp, like a knife piercing through my left ear and eye. Eventually, as I opened to that sharpness, the sensation shape-shifted into pulses. Then, gradually, even those pulses dissipated. Only then could I locate the pain in the lower-left quadrant of my mouth and eventually trace it to one particular tooth. Each pulsation gave way into another field of movement as I responded to my sensing, opening and shifting … and eventually, even the pain inside the tooth gave way.

Until then, I had never thought of these blindfolded experiments as anything but experiments in perception. At that point, however, I suddenly recognized the influence it had on pain—and, potentially, healing. I still did not understand why it had that effect. Whenever I sensed myself from the inside out as movements within movements, I noticed that I felt tremendous aliveness and freedom.

I was stunned. What had seemed relatively fixed and solid—my very own body—turned out to be interpenetrating movement. The shape and intensity and rhythm of the pulse would change and even disappear at times. I could sense many movements. Sometimes the rhythms were unstable and chaotic. Other times they would act like an orchestra—coherent and coordinated. Soon I discovered that my sensing was becoming attuned to these different rhythms. The movement became more coherent. What had seemed like an orchestra tuning up before a show, simultaneously and discordantly, had turned into music in its own right.

A deeply perceptive man, Jacques Lusseyran, wrote of a similar discovery of somatic awareness in his book, *And There Was Light*. In a chapter called "The Experience of Touch in Blindness" he said:

When I had eyes, my fingers used to be stiff, half dead at the ends of my hands, good only for picking up things. But now each one of them started out on its own. They explored things separately, changed levels, and, independently of each other, made themselves heavy or light.

Movement of fingers was terribly important, and had to be uninterrupted because objects do not stand at a given point, fixed there, confined to one form. They are alive, even the stones. What is more they vibrate and tremble. My fingers felt the pulsation distinctly, and if they failed to answer with a pulsation of their own, the fingers immediately became helpless and lost their sense of touch. But when they went toward things, in sympathetic vibration with them, they recognized them right away.

Yet there was something still more important than movement, and that was pressure. If I put my hand on the table without pressing it, I knew the table was there, but knew nothing about it. To find out, my fingers had to bear down, and the amazing thing is that the pressure was answered by the table at once. Being blind I thought I should have to go out to meet things, but I found that they came to me instead. I have never had to go more than halfway, and the universe became the accomplice of all my wishes.

If my fingers pressed the roundness of an apple, each one with a different weight, very soon I could not tell whether it was the apple or my fingers which were heavy. I didn't even know whether I was touching it or it was touching me. As I became part of the apple, the apple became part of me. And that was how I came to understand the existence of things.[6]

Now, bedridden and suffering from internal injuries, as I looked back on that experience of teaching the blind, it occurred to me that the lessons I had learned there might offer a pathway out of pain now. So rather than attempting to escape from the pain, I began to "sense" inside the sensation of pain. And in doing that, I realized that the pain was not fixed and immutable. Rather, I could feel waves moving through my organs and tissues.

As I sensed movement through my tissues, they responded to my sensing, the way a plant responds to sunlight: form and structure opening into the vast light of awareness. As space opened to me, I no longer felt pressure from pain, eventually diffusing entirely. I began to sense myself not as a solid body at all, but as movement within movements.

However, when I started to rise from bed in order to physically move around in space, the pain and bleeding often returned. This showed me that I needed to learn to rise up and move through the world with the same fluidity that I had discovered while resting.

As I began the practice of observing myself in order to understand and build on what worked, I learned how to use the pain and related sensations as feedback, helping me sense in real time how consciousness was organizing this community of cells. One thing I kept rediscovering was my habit of tensing up, and how this tension manifested in my daily-life activities in a myriad of ways. I realized that while this tensing or "contraction" might have begun as early attempts to help or protect me, in actuality it now had the opposite effect. As I opened to this realization, I began to see that my ability to get past the pain was not due to any "efforting" but rather to sensing my connection to something much larger. I came to realize that what truly helps is going beyond the limiting images, habits, and conditioning of the past. In the immediate experience of sensing, there was nothing above or below this vastness; there was nothing "other." There were only interpenetrating movements through which this "wholeness" renewed itself. I later came to call this expression of gratefulness for receiving the infinite—this "kissing back"—*presencing*.

The Healing Power of Presencing

Learning a new way to sense myself involved just a small shift in awareness. But it was enough not only to change my state of consciousness but also to reverse the progression of my dis-ease. That is, it was not just my perception of my body that changed; it was also my actual physiology. My whole system began to function differently. Healing and regeneration occurred.

This way of functioning—rather than being merely a fleeting relief from pain—gradually became a new way of living, a way that healed and renewed me. This mode of awareness—this ability to sense myself somatically, at a process level, in the bubbling, bursting, blooming of life—was the foundation of my complete recovery. Over time, I even started menstruating again. And years later I conceived naturally and enjoyed a wonderful pregnancy and ecstatic birth at home. Later, I came to teach what I had learned, as a self-sustaining process for transformative learning and change that anyone could adopt.

While I would never wish my traumatic experience on anyone else, at this point I am immensely grateful to have gone through it. Because what I learned from it was not just a matter of recovering from an illness. It was a turning point, an entry into a whole new way of being. As you move through this book I encourage you to reclaim your birthright: the gift of being embodied into the most finely tuned feedback system imaginable.

Just think, you were born into a body that—far from being a machine that wears down, assailed by the ravages of circumstance and time—is a supremely conducive environment for learning to live in the present moment, to sense and move with the flow of what is. This living, everchanging responsiveness of the body to awareness is the key to transformative learning and change. Embodying mindfulness takes us beyond the limited way in which we have known ourselves up to now—a way that we mistook for the ground of reality—then we get to discover and even create a whole new reality.

This new mode of functioning awakens us to the amazing self-sensing, self-organizing, and self-renewing system that we are. It promises us a revolution in self-discovery. The art and practice of Somatic Learning frees us to invent and discover a new realm of possibility, far beyond our wildest dreams.

While this experience of personal healing was profound, so too has been the process of sharing with students discoveries about the extraordinary capacities of somatic intelligence—in healing and awakening. What I had discovered was the fundamental role of awareness in shaping our experience, indeed our very aliveness. That "determining" role was not exclusive to one activity or another. Rather, I found that it underlies all activities—from the most common daily work, to the way we practice meditation or yoga, to how we converse with people. It is reflected in all our ways of evaluating meaning—electro-chemically, neuro-muscularly, sensing, feeling, thinking, anticipating, remembering, environing, etc.[7] As a result, I brought these insights into my practice as:

- a somatic psychotherapist
- a practitioner of various methods of touchwork
- a practitioner and teacher of meditation and yoga, expressive movement and dance
- a facilitator of dialogue as a form of social meditation
- a poet, writer, and performer.

All these practices proved fruitful disciplines for awakening somatic intelligence. Each provided a unique portal for deepening the inquiry.

As I began to teach, I discovered that anyone can learn to participate in the present, in the process of their own becoming, in a way that heals and transforms them. Rather than attempting to avoid pain, compensating for our weaknesses, or trying to accommodate some limitation or trauma— thus making ourselves smaller—we can actually do the inverse. We can use our circumstances to open us to something larger than we ever imagined. I feel such gratefulness for the gifts of awakening that these challenges have brought to our lives—as so many of my students have come to express. You will find some of their inspirational stories, told in their own words, throughout this book, scattered like breadcrumbs along a pathless path.

As pain and more obvious limitations disappear, the question becomes: what can we do to enhance our enjoyment of life?

Is it possible that even the slightest shift in awareness can bring about such profound change that we no longer live in the same body or even the same universe?

What if the most important change we can make for our health and liberation is the same?

What if liberation required no effort or act of will?

Somatic Learning represents an intersection between the practical and profound. It is an invitation into a deeper alignment with our innate intelligence. This intelligence brings about a self-sustainable new order that functions from these three fundamental characteristics: It is self-sensing, self-organizing, and self-renewing.

Larry's Story: Multi-Generational Healing

I had two missing discs and three collapsed vertebrae that were pinching the corresponding nerves. The symptoms were a constant tingling or numbness in my arms.

This was probably due to over-exercise (I did a tremendous amount of waterskiing, which compresses your whole skeleton). Other accidents may have also played a part. For example, in one snow-skiing accident I broke three ribs and collapsed a lung.

I had seen two physiatrists, who sent me to see two different surgeons. The surgeons told me I would lose the use of my arms if I did not have the collapsed vertebrae fused. In the surgery, they would cut me open through the front, spread my rib cage apart, move my esophagus to the side, and then screw in a couple of stainless steel plates between the vertebrae. Then they would take bone from elsewhere in my body and insert that into the space between the plates to start fusing the vertebrae together. When they were done they would staple me back together, and with a little bit of luck one would still have a voice. But once you fuse those vertebrae, you put more pressure on the vertebrae on either side of the fusion and you lose a lot of flexibility. This would ultimately lead to more problems later on. It didn't seem like a great idea, but they said there was no other way to save my arms.

A consultant to the high-tech company where I was the CEO saw me without my brace one day and asked if my neck was getting better. I replied, "No, in fact the opposite, but since I'm now going to schedule the surgery, I've given up wearing the neck brace, which wasn't helping anyway." He encouraged me to see Dr. Kaparo before I went in for the surgery … so I did.

After a few sessions with her, my neck and arms were much better, and I had greatly increased flexibility. I was able to maintain this progress by taking about five minutes a day to do the "standing pour forward" and a "quick spinal release" both in the morning and right before bed. Soon the sensations in my arms went away entirely, and I never had to get the surgery.

Occasionally, when I drove my racecars, I would aggravate my neck again and some tingling would return. But I could get myself back on track going to see Dr. Kaparo and just practicing those two exercises.

I began to wonder if Dr. Kaparo could help my wife, a schoolteacher, who had been suffering from daily migraines for many years. The irony is that my wife had been diligently working to improve her fitness and health by working with a personal trainer. As it turned out, much of what she did actually exacerbated her chronic tension. It wasn't long after my wife started to see Dr. Kaparo and modify her normal workout, in addition to incorporating the spinal elongation and awareness practices that she learned, that her headaches almost vanished completely.

We decided to bring our daughters to Dr. Kaparo. One had suffered from spondylosis and had to drop out of school from time to time because it was impossible for her to function, much less focus under so much pain. Again, we saw miraculous improvement immediately.

Our other daughter had worn leg braces for years as a young child to address a pronounced pigeon-toe problem. When the braces didn't work to correct her legs, we were guided to have her practice figure skating as a remedy, which she did for years … again with little improvement. In just one session with Dr. Kaparo, we could see a marked improvement in her legs and in her lower back.

Over the years we have seen so many people we referred improve their health through Somatic Learning.

Be a Light Unto Yourself
   —*The Buddha's last words*

CHAPTER 2

Fundamental Principles of Somatic Learning: The Science and Practice of Awakening Somatic Intelligence

Conventionally people regard "practice" as a process through which they will eventually acquire a skill or result. While this certainly has limited value, in the current context "practice" is not about efforting toward an accomplishment in time, but rather begins from the "result level"—meaning that this intelligence is available here and now. We are simply learning to "drop into it," to allow it to reveal itself, so that whatever we participate in arises as an expression of this intelligence, right now. This can be seen as the "ultimate practice," embracing whatever is arising through our full embodiment. As we "drink in" the infinite, we presence or "take up" vast spaciousness, infusing our whole being with the consciousness that pervades all of existence. And as we "kiss back," our heartfelt savoring overflows, embuing this spaciousness with the luminosity of love. This ecstatic "practice" refers to the deepening of our capacity to bear the infinite as the beloved, as intimately as our breath, bones, blood.

This nondual awareness can express itself in every aspect of living. The term "nondual" (meaning "not two") is used to denote affinity, or unity, in contrast to duality, separateness, or multiplicity. It refers to the idea that things can appear distinct while not being separate.

When one engages somatic intelligence, one awakens to compassion, peace, and happiness as self-sustaining modes of living.

One unique contribution this book makes is in exploring the implications of this embodied mindfulness for healing. Somatic Learning can be used as a skillful means to transform pain, stress, trauma, and even aging. This book will show you how to utilize somatic intelligence—your own inner guidance system—as a compass to navigate the conditioned aspects of experience from a state of limitless awareness. For example, in addressing back pain, the approach of conventional medicine attempts to resolve the problem through mechanical exercise, surgery, or medication in an effort to eliminate the unwanted, localized sensations of pain. From the perspective of Somatic Learning, as you begin to utilize feeling and sensation as feedback, you become an open, learning-oriented system. You become more self-sensing and self-organizing, transforming your structure and functioning in a way that eases the pressure and allows the organism to follow its own natural course toward healing and self-renewal, so there is no problem to fix. The process functions at the "result level" from the beginning. As you embody greater freedom and aliveness, all movement—in space (such as walking, running, bending, lifting) as well as intrinsic movements (such as in sitting, standing, lying)—can function without strain. In this way, the "dangerous opportunity" of back pain becomes a laboratory for deepening presence—for being an expression of infinite intelligence.

Instead of following a teaching, or method, or lineage, Somatic Learning is a way of embodying and expressing somatic intelligence—so you can become, in the words of Buddha, "a Light unto yourself." Unbounded intelligence lives in you as you, and in this intimate dance with life, you and the infinite are one. It is not "about" you and yet, there could be nothing more "personal," in the sense of most deeply felt and articulated through the unique way your embodiment sources the infinite, and all the conditions that arise within it—excluding nothing. "We have never touched like this before."[1]

This chapter integrates research and concepts from many fields of science, psychology, and spiritual discipline to render the process of change less esoteric and more knowable. Understanding fundamental principles such as embodied mindfulness, differentiation, presencing, proprioception, interoception, neuroplasticity, learning and habituation cycles will provide a conceptual basis for utilizing the practices in the book to enhance happiness, love, and healthy longevity and deliver you from pain, stress, trauma, and degenerative aging.

In teaching, I start by conducting people into a Somatic Meditation, and then explore the conceptual and scientific basis, always referring back to their own direct experience. In book form, it feels necessary to attempt this unfolding in reverse. Although the concepts that follow may seem abstract at first, they can serve as reference points to deepen your embodiment of the results when you begin the actual practices. Even as I write about concepts, I will continually point your attention back to how the ideas can inform your own direct experience.

Given the subject/object structure of our language, it is particularly difficult to speak from a nondual perspective. Since the principles are meant to point to the unknowable or ineffable, not to the known, you may feel confused at times. As you read this chapter, I invite you to suspend judgment or the need "to know" in the usual sense, and to trust what happens without trying to grasp after meaning. In the beginning this may feel awkward, even frustrating to your need to nail something down, to render it understandable. But presencing requires a living into the unknown, relaxed and curious, without efforting to grasp anything. If I place a flower in your hand, your hand must stay open in order to perceive its beauty. If it closes in around it, the gift of its beauty will be lost to you. Your fingers must stay open to dialogue with the flower, to know it and be known. Similarly, remain receptively open as you sense fluctuations in the bodymind, and release the struggle to "wrap your mind around something"—this will open a portal to direct perception of the true nature of reality.

> You must know for yourself, directly, the truth of yourself and
> you cannot realize it through another, however great. There is no
> authority that can reveal it.
> —*J. Krishnamurti*[2]

Neuroplasticity

Since it is mindful awareness itself that transforms conditions of the bodymind, we must carefully develop this art and practice. Current research on neuroplasticity verifies that "you can use your mind to change your brain," producing not just short-term effects but long-term, permanent changes, since "neurons that fire together, wire together" (in the famous words of the Canadian psychologist Donald Hebb).[3] Then the brain's more integrated intelligent functioning changes how the mind responds to the circumstances and conditions of life. As the neural substrate is enhanced, it supports neural functioning that increases our ability to express and embody somatic intelligence. Further, research shows that awareness transforms the bodymind in the direction of optimal, coherent functioning. This represents an evolutionary shift from *surviving* to *thriving.*

> Recent studies of mindfulness practices reveal that they can result
> in profound improvements in a range of physiological, mental,

and interpersonal domains of our lives. Cardiac, endocrine, and immune functions are improved with mindfulness practices. Empathy, compassion, and interpersonal sensitivity seem to be improved. People who come to develop the capacity to pay attention in the present moment without grasping onto their inevitable judgments also develop a deeper sense of well-being and what can be considered a form of mental coherence.

—*Daniel J. Siegel, MD*[4]

We are the fruits of three and a half billion years of evolution. Evolutionary biology has made us far more prone to fear than to contentment. Being vigilant to recognize potential dangers has had tremendous biological advantage. It keeps us alert to threats. The worst it does for us is produce anxiety and stress. But if we miss a possible danger, we may not continue to live at all.

Recent studies have shown that we are far more trainable toward helplessness and despair than toward responsibility and freedom. This underscores the importance of ongoing practice to prepare the body-mind to presence happiness, love, embodied joy, and aliveness in a more deeply integrated way. As the research confirms, when you stimulate the neural networks of positive states you gradually strengthen them. By predisposing the brain toward joy, we are learning to be happy from the inside out.

Embodied Mindfulness

Research has shown that the more a person is aware of their own body, the more their insula lights up in an MRI. The more active their insula is, the more empathic they are to other people, which is the foundation of compassion and loving kindness.

—*Drs. Rick Hanson and Richard Mendius*[5]

Since mindfulness activates the insula, the part of your brain responsible for awareness of the internal state of your body, it follows that awakening somatic intelligence is especially useful in engaging the insula.

It may prove helpful to understand how the insula and "mirror neurons" are involved in empathy. To quote Drs. Hanson and Mendius again:

> When a person you are observing is experiencing a deep feeling, some of the same cells in your insula activate that activate when you yourself are feeling that feeling. This way, you get a sense from the inside-out of what the other person is going through. There may be as much as ten percent of the neurons that are involved in any of your own internal sensations that get involved when you observe somebody in the same state.[6]

The relevance of these findings to emotional and social intelligence, attachment behavior, and interpersonal neurobiology is readily apparent. The implications of awakening somatic intelligence are practical, pervasive, and profound, as recent brain research clearly demonstrates. There is a high correlation between interoception (awareness of your internal state), empathy, heightened immune function, and a sense of well-being.

Drs. Rick Hanson and Richard Mendius continue:

> Meditation also trains the brain to enter and sustain happy states of being. It leads the hypothalamus and the brain stem to reward the rest of the brain with pleasant hormones, like oxytocin, and neurotransmitters like dopamine and norepinephrine. All of this establishes positive internal states that become increasingly important goals that the brain, and thus the mind, increasingly inclines itself toward. It's like you are training your own brain to lean increasingly toward happiness.[7]

The Gift of Embodiment

How can we enhance our happiness and enjoyment of life? Often we think of enjoyment as coming from outside ourselves, as someone or something that brings joy to us. But I am speaking here of what arises in awareness.

We are taking in the infinite with each breath. All the stars, everything in the known universe, have contributed to the air that we breathe.

Take a deep breath. What happens as you savor it? As you extend your sensing into the space where you and the infinite converge, does your experience become more delicious?

Presencing is a way of leaning into the beloved, as a cat will sometimes lean into the stroking. We hear the enjoyment expressed in the purring. When you lean into it, can you sense it more deeply?

Somatic Learning provides a discipline for a new participation in life. It is a practice for awakening to who we really are by receiving the gift of our embodiment—not what we mistake for our "body" as "object," but as the embodiment of spaciousness in the actual blooming of life, in the here and now.

The practice is one of tasting the moment, to sense what arises in the present and to learn to extend our sensing, to lean into it, to savor it. When we sense the edge of our known world, we can extend presence to receive the infinite opening beyond and through the known, as we might follow the ringing of a temple bell. Your listening can extend as far as the vibration travels, moving through the wood and glass of the meditation hall, beyond the rosemary bushes and over the rolling hills. You can extend your presence beyond the known boundaries of ordinary experience and continue to open infinitely; no longer delineating where the sound ends and the silence begins. So too, with the unbounded consciousness that you are.

The following excerpt by Matthew Sanford, a man paralyzed from an accident since he was thirteen years of age, beautifully demonstrates the efficacy of a mindful awareness practice in awakening somatic intelligence.

> I struggled to believe that I could actually feel the inner energetic sensations.... When I look at my legs, when I consider what's missing—voluntary movement, muscle tone, flexion—what is it that remains? Obviously, my legs are still physically present in the same way that a table is present. But what else? I do experience this new level of sensation, but it's not like

normal sensation. It is not immediately responsive; for example, when I pinch my leg, shock waves do not instantly invade my brain. The truth is that my legs are not very interested in what surrounds them, in the texture of my pants, in the softness of my socks. Instead, they present a hum, an energetic buzz. (Imagine the buzz you feel after you finally get into bed after an exhausting day.) It gets louder sometimes, tingles sometimes, even seems to change its "color" when my legs get cold. Moreover, this buzz is directly affected by the quality of my perception, by how well I listen. Meditative attention amplifies it to the point of exaggeration; an engaging social interaction pushes it into the distant background; a rock concert makes it disappear completely.

And yet, this energetic buzz persists, fluctuates, moves, and spreads. It also reflects changes in my bodily state. For example, it becomes agitated if my bladder is too full, or if my bowels need emptying. It spikes during systemic pain, like when I have a high fever. More important for my yoga, this energetic awareness responds to my mind's intent. It becomes louder when my physical body comes into greater alignment and is "darkened" in places within my body that my mind has unknowingly abandoned.

… when I truly listen, I hear what exists before movement. Through paralysis, the outer layer of my legs and torso have been stripped away. What remains is what's present before I enter the world through effort and action, before I engage my will. I begin to perceive the history of my body as similar to the fate of an artichoke as we eat it. Green leaf after green leaf, thriving muscle after thriving muscle, is peeled away until nothing but the heart remains—a heart that presents itself first as silence.

I received something in exchange for absorbing so much trauma at age thirteen. I experience a more direct contact with an inner presence of consciousness—the heart of the artichoke. Although my life has taken much away, it has also revealed a powerful insight.[8]

When you take the opportunity of experiencing "what is" as "gift," despite apparent limitations, physical or otherwise, you meet the present fully. With awakened somatic intelligence, your presence can dimensionally extend to become a co-creative participant in the "quantum coherence" of "all that is."

Where do we start? It begins with our own immediate felt-sense of receiving the unbounded spaciousness, as close as the breath, and as immediate. When we embody mindfulness, the infinite or nondual awareness is grounded in the intimacy of our own direct experiencing. The conditional referents of experience—sensations, feelings, and thoughts—are sensed as expressions of the non-conditional, co-arising. Like the tiny boats painted at the outer edge of a Zen scroll, they point to the infinite. In this way, the misidentification of taking "image/object" consciousness for the ground of reality is recognized and transformed.

When we receive the gift of our embodiment in the most finely tuned feedback system, the human organism, our natural state of joyous well-being is reclaimed. When somatic intelligence awakens, the inherent wisdom of the embodied mindfulness, which is self-sensing, self-organizing, and self-renewing, becomes obvious. Embodied mindfulness unfolds as the perfect learning environment for presencing the joy of being fully alive in the freedom-streaming spaciousness.

Proprioception

Proprioception is, literally, how we "sense ourselves." There are three main sources of input into our proprioceptive system. One of them, *kinesthesia,* is the feeling of movement derived from all skeletal and muscular structures. Kinesthesia also includes the feeling of pain, our orientation in space, the passage of time, and rhythm. A second source, *visceral feedback,* consists of the miscellaneous impressions from our internal organs. *Labyrinthine or vestibular feedback*—the feeling of balance as related to our position in space—is provided by the cochlea, an organ of the inner ear.

In the beginning, before we emerge from the amniotic waters, movement is perception. To the fetus floating within the womb, the development of the senses and the perceptions are not separate from the development of movement."

—*Louise Steinman*[9]

The physiological term "proprioception" refers to the ability to sense, evaluate, and respond to stimuli sensed by the proprioceptors, actual nerves embedded in our tissues (muscles, joints, and tendons). These cells constantly communicate with the brain, orienting the body to its movement, position, and tone. It is our sixth sense. The other five senses provide information about the outer world. Proprioception provides information about the inner world, which we alone inhabit. Physicist David Bohm used the term "proprioceptive intelligence" to describe an optimal state of self-sensing, self-correcting, and self-organizing awareness—allowing for coherent participation in life through the integral functioning of all modes of intelligence.

In contrast, when we rely almost exclusively on visual perception, it is easy to become identified with the three-dimensional reality that we see. For instance, we mistake what we see in the mirror at three feet away for what is going on "here" at no distance. Without the integration of somatic intelligence, we invariably become identified with this image of ourselves and reduce ourselves to living out of that image-bound reality. This is in contrast to the freedom and aliveness inherent in how life senses itself from the inside out, at no distance, as the bubbling, bursting, blooming forth of consciousness in the here and now.

Even as people begin their somatic practice, they often rely on visual perception where it is not effective. Instead of proprioception (sensing), they will create an image of themselves that they try to move or affect—from the outside in. This further perpetuates the fragmentation of mind and "body," compounding the problems that arose from that fragmentation in the first place.

Matthew Sanford again:

Just doing four poses was exciting enough. My body, paralyzed though it was, was taking the shapes of real, bona fide yoga poses. I would sit on the floor, use my arms to move my legs, bring the soles of my feet together, grab underneath them, and lift my chest. The outward result was pleasing. If a snapshot of my version of baddha konasana were held up next to a snapshot of another beginning student's pose, they would have looked roughly the same. I could do it.

For many students, this is as far as they delve into the heart of yoga. They practice the poses in a strictly physical manner. They access only the poses' outline, using their bodies to fulfill the intended shape. For them, yoga is similar to gymnastics or acrobatics—that is, an expression of their outer body.

In my practice, I encountered the same limitation within my paralyzed body. When I did a pose, I would typically feel the muscles in my upper body straining and working. But my lower body remained essentially quiet. What cues I experienced came from my physical position, for example, from the shift in balance between having my legs straight and having them bent. In short, my perception traveled primarily from outside to in.

The feeling is similar to looking at your image in a full-length mirror. You can become so fixated on this outer image that you briefly lose connection to the "inside" of the figure in front of you. Perhaps you go to straighten the knee in the picture and are surprised when you realize that it is your knee that is straightening. Now imagine living with access only to the image in the mirror, that is, without the feeling of having your knee straighten. In some ways, that is what it is like to be paralyzed. Moreover, that was how I felt when I did a yoga pose—my lower body was only an image.

But then something changed. My yoga poses gained a measure of inward, three-dimensional depth and did so without flexing muscles. A sense of energy awakened not just within my unparalyzed body, but even more profoundly through the silence of my paralyzed body.[10]

As Lusseyran's and Sanford's descriptions so beautifully articulate, even in situations of "disability" or, perhaps, especially so (an idea we will explore in Chapter 5 in the Spindrift research), the darkness can "light up." The "enlightenment" or "proprioceptive illumination" (described in more detail later in this chapter) represents an awakening of somatic intelligence. This awakening serves as a portal into a new realm of possibility—a rabbit hole into the wonderland of a self-sensing, self-organizing, and self-renewing universe that is immediately apprehensible.

The Primacy of Perception and Beliefs: A New Biology

Biologists are beginning to address the phenomenon of perception, or inner conscious awareness, as a primary causative reality. I refer you here to Bruce Lipton's work as one of the leading exponents of the New Biology, a field of research that defies the "old" biology's belief in the primacy of genes as the determinant of what we become.[11] In contrast, the new biology offers us the field of Epigenetics, which recognizes the primacy of perception and belief in determining how our genes participate in what we become. Our genome is not our destiny; only an indicator. The new biology is an epistemological science by necessity (it takes into consideration our meaning-making). It is a science that does not dismiss how we make meaning from "reality" but sees ourselves as meaning-makers participating in creating the reality we perceive.

In *The Biology of Belief,* Bruce Lipton shows how our beliefs form our biology. He gives several examples that seem especially relevant to our practice. In India, when elephants are very young, one leg is tied up with a small rope to a tree or pole. The young elephant struggles for a few days trying to get loose but soon recognizes the futility of this struggle and stops trying to fight the rope. A belief is now installed that "I can't get loose when a rope is tied to my leg." As the elephant grows, that programmed belief continues to operate, so that even when the elephant is full grown and more than capable of taking down the pole or tree and ripping apart the rope, it will stop even trying to get loose as soon as a rope is tied to a leg.

When we are very young, our subconscious minds are programmed like the elephant's by those around us. Our brain functions primarily in theta, delta, and alpha states until we are five or six years old. In other words, we live in a more or less hypnotic state, primarily suitable for absorbing programs rather than conscious thinking in these early years. And like the elephant, these early programs continue to be what operates even when they are clearly obsolete or in conflict with the intentions or perceptions of our conscious mind.

> The past is not dead. In fact, it is not even past.
> —*William Faulkner, novelist*

It is important here to remember that the conscious mind utilizes a small part of the brain (primarily the pre-frontal cortex) and is capable of processing approximately 40 bits of information per second, whereas the subconscious mind utilizes the remainder of the brain, processing approximately 40 *million* bits of information per second. That is, it processes a million times more information per second than the conscious brain. This explains why what is programmed into it has a much more powerful influence generally on our biology and our lives than what we think consciously.

Lipton provides us with another story to exemplify how this works. Maybe you've seen a stage hypnotist ask someone in a trance state to lift a glass of water off the table after giving them the suggestion that the glass weighs a ton. You can see the person struggling and straining, attempting to lift the glass, but he cannot. While the mind of the hypnotized person is activating the muscles involved in lifting, it is also simultaneously activating muscles that resist the lift, which reflects his belief that the glass is extremely heavy. His subconscious mind is orchestrating this very complex set of activities that creates a reality coherent with his belief. Both sets of muscles are working all out to handle this glass, like an isometric exercise, so there is no net effect on the glass. In this way whatever beliefs we acquire will shape our biology.

Therefore, it behooves us to uncover the beliefs that we have been programmed with before our own conscious thought processes developed and to update or replace them with beliefs that are more relevant and congruent with our conscious thoughts and intentions.

The Old Paradigm. Many of us may have experienced some kind of trauma (from our early childhood, as well as in our pre- or peri-natal stages of development) through attachment patterns that have installed certain beliefs particular to us as individuals. However, most of our programming arises from collective beliefs of what we might call consensual reality (what we agree within a given paradigm to accept as "real"). Let's explore a few of the beliefs of the prevailing old paradigm that may still function as ropes around our leg now.

1. We function as relatively fixed objects.
2. We are separate from everything else.
3. Gravity is a force that needs to be overcome by effort.

These beliefs are based on the reductionism, materialism, and determinism of the socially prevailing scientific paradigm arising from Aristotelian thinking and Newtonian physics. However, in the latter half of the twentieth century, scientists and philosophers postulated a new paradigm, articulated in quantum physics and a philosophy of wholism.

The New Paradigm. Let's consider a few new beliefs that may be more relevant and empowering than those of the old paradigm.

1. We function as self-sensing, self-organizing, and self-renewing energy beings.
2. We are interconnected with all that is.
3. Gravity provides an opportunity to sense and liberate us from our patterns of habitual tension.

The art and practice of Somatic Learning optimally supports the full embodiment of the quality commonly referred to as "mindfulness" in our lives through awakening somatic intelligence. It develops an open dialogue between the conscious and subconscious parts of our mind. This dialogue allows what we sense in the immediacy of our silent level of experience to influence and update our beliefs.

As we sense the feedback arising from the bodymind and gravity throughout our organism, we learn new ways of functioning that are congruent with non self-limiting beliefs. The old programmed responses are erased, and our habitual tensions release into a more enlivened and integrated functioning. Through the Somatic Meditations we develop a more highly differentiated response-ability. This enhanced capacity for self-sensing, self-organizing (self-correcting), and self-renewing is the hallmark of the practice of Somatic Learning.

Presencing—Embodying the Infinite

As we clear the old programming and learn to live into the unknown, the infinite reveals itself to us so that we come to know it intimately. I refer to this process of living into the unknown and embodying it as presencing. With each breath, we can feel the infinite coming to us freely, effortlessly, as we open to it. We drink it in, riding the waves of our joy and interest. We are not simply growing more of the same, there is a transformative change from this interpenetration with the infinite. I often describe this as the convergence of rivers, the way two currents will interpenetrate and form a new streaming of life. A whole new emergence occurs that did not previously exist. This new life displays the three attributes of somatic intelligence: it is self-sensing, self-organizing, and self-renewing.

Only what grows out of your direct experiencing has the power to change everything. Since the "body "and the "world" live in your experience ... not the reverse as is generally conceived ... how you open to receive experience will change how the bodymind unfolds in the present as form, sensations, chemistry, feeling, thinking, memory and anticipation: the biology of becoming.

Neither presencing nor differentiation, the two primary processes of Somatic Learning, involve efforting. In fact, they clearly demonstrate that you can't get "here" from "there." In ordinary (image/object-bound) experience, we just keep trying harder ... efforting, straining, tensing toward accomplishment. When we truly recognize the futility of this, the efforting ceases, and a portal opens into deeper listening. From this deeper and somatic (here-now, all-at-once, at-no-distance) feeling/sensing/knowing, our presence extends beyond the limitations of the familiar world into new dimensions of consciousness. Movement responds according to how we sense it. As the study of quantum mechanics has revealed, nature behaves according to how we probe it. The classic example is light. Light is neither a wave nor a particle. It reveals itself according to how we form an experiment.

Likewise, the immediate feedback we receive from being embodied is continually responding to how we perceive ourselves. Our organismic functioning reflects our state of consciousness. This reveals the beauty of Somatic Meditations. We can see the participation of our thoughts or state of consciousness in how our "body" responds. Those of us who have meditated have likely experienced how easily we can get lost in thought when we are "trying" to meditate and not even realize it until we are at the tail end of a long stream of thought. In the same way we can feel trapped, as though in a relatively fixed "object-level body," by the limitations of identification.

> Fear drives us to shine a focused beam of light onto what we think we must know, to keep us safe, to give us a sense of truth, of keeping the world the way we think it should be. We have words and ideas that frame and form the field of awareness that dull our senses, shaping what we think we know, in thoughts, about what can be known. But the real truth is that those 'cognitive contraptions' help structure a neural attempt to make sense of a complex world, only to then entrap us in the very structures that we have created.
>
> —Daniel J. Siegel, MD[12]

Anything we do to try to correct the problems that our limited state of consciousness creates, at the same level of identification at which the problems formed (i.e., relating to one's "body" as though it were a relatively fixed, three-dimensional object), will merely perpetuate the problem and add more complexity to it. Just as Einstein pointed out … "The significant problems we face cannot be solved at the same level of thinking we were at when we created them."[13]

Somatic Learning is not about fixing problems, which perpetuates the same fragmentation from which the problems arose in the first place. The intention of the practice is awakening. Awareness lights up our state of consciousness, the processes of thought and feeling (conscious and subconscious) that underlie the problems as they are reflected through the "body." Somatic Learning is the art and practice of awakening the natural wisdom of embodied mindfulness, the intelligence of the living which Nora and James Oschman refer to as a "veritable symphony of vibratory messages." According to their continuum communication model, these messages:

> … travel to and fro, alerting each part of the organism about the activities taking place in each other part. What we refer to as "consciousness" is the totality of these vibrations. Disease, disorder, and pain arise within portions of the vibratory continuum where information flows are restricted. Restrictions occur locally because infections, physical injury, and emotional trauma alter properties of the fabric.
>
> The living matrix retains a record or memory of the influences that have been exerted upon it. When vibrations pass through tissues, they are altered by the signatures of the stored information. In this way, our consciousness and our choices are influenced by memories stored in soft tissues.[14]

Yet, because somatic intelligence is self-sensing, self-organizing, and self-renewing, the residue of pain and trauma needn't determine our experience of ourselves and what we become. Somatic intelligence liberates us from bondage to the past, including the limitation of our genes, as well as from early trauma, giving way to greater freedom and aliveness.

As our awareness is liberated through Somatic Learning, a new world of possibilities opens up to us.

Awareness is the function of isolating "new" sensory-motor phenomena in order to learn to recognize and control them. It is only through the exclusionary function of awareness that the involuntary is made voluntary, the unknown is made known, and the never-done is made doable. Awareness serves as a probe, recruiting new material for the repertoire of voluntary consciousness.

The upshot of this is somatic learning begins by focusing awareness on the unknown. This active focusing identifies traits of the unknown that can be associated with traits already known in one's conscious repertoire. Through this process the unknown becomes known by the voluntary consciousness. In a word, the unlearned becomes learned.

—*Thomas Hanna*[15]

Differentiation

How does somatic awakening occur? One way is through a process of differentiation. By differentiation, I mean simply noticing change or movement. When you differentiate awareness, what you experienced previously as solid and relatively fixed, like "the body" or "the ground," will now reveal itself as ever-changing, movement within movement. Each time you learn to differentiate more, the edge of the known changes. It is like falling deeper and deeper through the rabbit hole, into a wonderland of possibility.

Eventually, it becomes absurd to mistake whatever you can sense/feel/know now as the ground of reality, as "the ground" keeps opening itself to you. You are standing on the threshold of the unbounded spaciousness, sensing the invitation to know it ever more deeply and intimately. Taking up that invitation, you actually extend your presence, creating a new edge between the known and the unknown. As you walk, you interpenetrate with the ground and with space, for instance. Like rivers converging, you are not only renewing and reorganizing yourself but the whole universe, as it opens infinitely to your touch, to being received by you. This is what I refer to as proprioceptive illumination.

Proprioceptive Illumination

This proprioceptive illumination lights up the edge—"where the two worlds meet" as Rumi would call it, the known and unknown. The sense of "self" inevitably becomes much more fluid, as awareness is no longer "image-bound." Each time you live into the unknown, you have a new perspective from which to perceive and re-cohere the known; your presence extends. So what is the self? Where is it located? Where does it start? Where does it stop? Eventually we see the "the self" as no more than a construct for a purpose, like a sand castle built at the edge of the sea. Whereas consciousness is like the sea itself. When we disenthrall, when we cease being captive to our fixation with the image of the "self," we find that we are the embodiment of unbounded consciousness.

Shosanah's Story: Ruby Slippers

Finding her way through the health concerns that she and her family have faced honed Shosanah into a sensitive and profound healer. Her influence has widened to include many people that she generously guides through both acute and chronic life challenges.

I found my way to Somatic Learning in search of help for my four-year-old son. After an intestinal crisis that led to exploratory surgery, he was diagnosed with an auto-immune disease. He continued to suffer bouts of enormous intestinal pain. Rather than accepting his diagnosis as a life sentence, I used the information from the tests and surgery to go my own way in search of wholeness through diet, cleansing, homeopathy, supplements, and hands-on healing. Beorn's challenges became a doorway into new worlds of possibility, which have in turn opened doors for many others. His diagnosis has long since become irrelevant. He is happy and vibrantly healthy. Somatic Learning has been an essential part of his healing.

Dr. Kaparo's work with Beorn extended far beyond his intestinal complaints. As a young child, he was reckless and daring, resulting in accidents and injuries. Many a time Dr. Kaparo helped to invite his bones, muscles, and ligaments back into alignment. Over time he grew wiser, and his coordination began to catch up with his adventuresome spirit. Now he combines art and athletics in bold new ways, such as riding his ripstick around while playing the violin.

In the first session with Beorn, Dr. Kaparo was able to listen with her hands and join with his inner intelligence to release tightened sphincters, ease his spasms, and begin the process of healing. As his pain eased, our family's relationship with Somatic Learning was born.

Beorn often needed help between sessions, and Dr. Kaparo agreed to teach me. I quickly learned that my greatest obstacle to co-creating healing with Beorn was the enormous accumulated tension in my own body, from years of severe scoliosis. In my twenties I had been told that

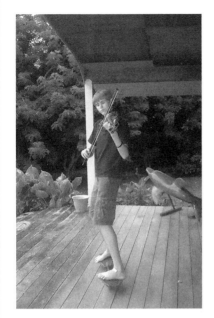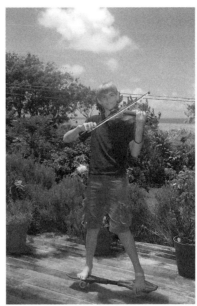

Beorn has benefitted from Somatic Learning.

it was too late to help my scoliosis. Three pregnancies compounded the problem. Despite having worked with many skilled therapists, by the time I started studying Somatic Learning in 2000, I lived in constant pain. Even lying on my back could create spasms. This began a long process of inner and outer dialogue, some of it on the table, and increasingly more of it through the Yoga of Somatic Learning. As my spine unwound, I grew in height. In my fifties I am a full inch taller than I was previously.

Creating new structure, an amazing and sometimes painful process, can often be less challenging than maintaining it. Once out of session and back in the stresses of life, my system would revert to its proprioceptive memory of curvature and misalignment, and pain would follow. The practice of Somatic Learning became a lifeline through which I learned to integrate—and more importantly to recreate—these changes.

Recently I've graduated to doing back bends, both from the floor and from the shoulder stand. As I prepare my pose, I rest upside down (fully inverted) on my shoulders, then one at a time (while remaining on my shoulders) I pour my legs out, bringing my feet to the floor behind me. The first time I attempted to move my legs toward the floor, I was filled with fear. But the first time my toe touched the floor I was in awe! Day by day, I travel further, surpassing old limits and discovering new worlds.

For me the gift is to travel with my awareness so deeply within my structure that I can initiate movement from the core of my being. My spine may revert to a familiar curve and the muscular tension reassert itself. But I can change that, in minutes, through breath, attention, and subtle movement. Now I can go beyond repair, to find space and movement that is completely new.

My healing journey was long because misalignment was my entire cellular memory. For most people the loss of height and freedom comes more gradually. Somatic Learning allows a path for discovering, retaining, and reclaiming that freedom.

Our tall, lean children started developing scoliosis as they grew. Fortunately, their practice of Somatic Learning changed the course of their genetic destiny. They each have a personal practice, and we also work together. Working with a partner who holds space for your energy to flow, or assists with the unwinding, is enormously helpful. As you discover new space and freedom, and learn to recreate it at will, there often follows an ability to help others achieve these same goals through facilitated yoga.

My daughter, Chanterelle, loves ballet. She has a natural grace, but the ballet poses easily pulled her developing spine out of alignment as she tried to match with her muscles what she studied with her eyes. Working with Dr. Kaparo, she learned to feel the poses and initiate movement from the center of her being, with attention and breath moving bones, with fascia and muscles joining the flow. The same pose or movement that had previously twisted and contorted her became a portal for lengthening, straightening, and undoing tension. As with yoga, the challenge with dance is that while one is learning to move from the core, it is difficult to move as quickly as traditional classes are taught, since they focus on rapid achievement of an outer form. For my family, the solution is often to take a break from classes while we integrate the inner work with the outer pose.

Three years ago Chanterelle fell in love with playing the piano. The somatic intelligence she had developed now manifested in an intrinsic ability to transcend the boundaries between body, fingers, mind, and instrument. She moves like a ballerina across the keys, music pouring from her heart though her hands, her body free of muscular tension.

The Yoga of Somatic Learning involves simultaneous travel on the inner and outer planes. The transformational magic that delights us cannot be achieved by tensing and stretching muscles. The doorway is through consciousness, breath, and elongation. The body is literally a portal to new universes: universes that have always been available to us, but which we have forgotten, or not yet learned to access. Consciousness becomes our ruby slippers. Awareness allows movement, which opens space for further travel of spirit and form. I am filled with gratitude for having learned and practiced this journey.

Right now as I speak to you, I cause fluctuations in the field of consciousness. These are non-material; you can't touch them, taste them, smell them, see them, because they are quantum-mechanical events. Just as an electron is a quantum of electricity and a photon a quantum of light, a thought, a flicker of intention is a quantum of consciousness. These quantum-mechanical events in consciousness become the flux of neuro-transmitters in my brain. They cause hormonal changes, they result in the transmission of neural impulses. They result in the vibration of vocal cords, the production of sound. All my feelings, all my emotions, all my desires, all my instincts, all my drives, every thought or urge I have, literally becomes a molecule. And that's how I construct my body, from consciousness.

—*Deepak Chopra*

CHAPTER 3

Engaging the Natural Wisdom of Embodied Mindfulness

Somatic Learning involves an open dialoguing between the sub-cortical and cortical parts of the nervous system—that is self-sensing and self-organizing and self-renewing. For instance, in walking I can mechanically locomote my "body as object" in discourse (a percussive back and forth) with the ground. In contrast, I can have an open dialogue with the ground in which I am self-organizing or learning from our convergence, subtly shape-shifting in response to the force of gravity drawing me to the center of the earth and the support rising from the ground as it breaks my fall.

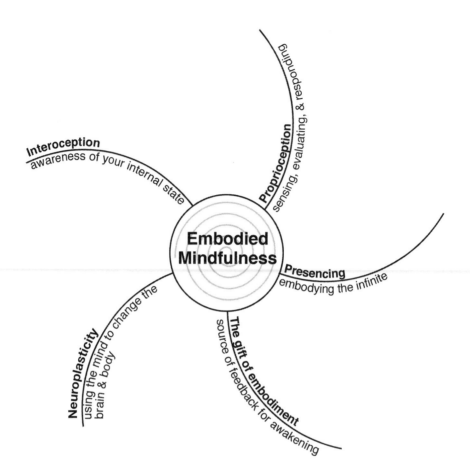

Interoception
awareness of your internal state

Proprioception
sensing, evaluating, & responding

Embodied Mindfulness

Presencing
embodying the infinite

Neuroplasticity
using the mind to change the brain & body

The gift of embodiment
source of feedback for awakening

I often ask people to walk barefoot across a streambed when I work with groups on retreat. It provides a context for discerning the difference between learning and habit systems in an immediately tangible way. If the habit cycle prevails, it can be quite painful, as you tense more to guard against discomfort. However, if the learning cycle prevails, if your system is responsive to your encounter with the ground, then even the pressure of jagged rocks can massage you, as though you've been touched all over. Your whole organism shape-shifts to accommodate the changing pressure. As you walk across the streambed, if you sense yourself and the ground connecting fluidly like two rivers converging, even in just a few steps, you will feel less dense, more relaxed and alert, and enjoy greater freedom and aliveness.

Cycles of Learning and Habituation

Habituation is a degenerative cycle, which occurs in a closed system, characterized by high tension, which leads to insensitivity, which leads to inefficient action, which leads to more insensitivity. The cycle is ultimately entropic. This is the cycle that we commonly witness and associate with aging. It reveals how our subconscious beliefs shape our biology.

Learning is a generative cycle, which requires an open system, characterized by minimal tension, which supports sensitivity, which supports efficient and intelligent action, which supports increasing sensitivity and awareness. This system is ultimately negentropic—it is evolutionary and intelligent—self-sensing, self-organizing, and self-renewing.

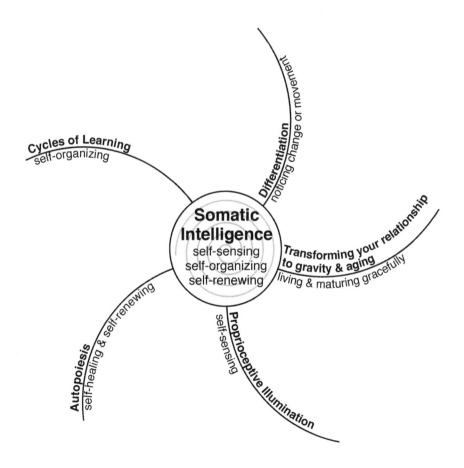

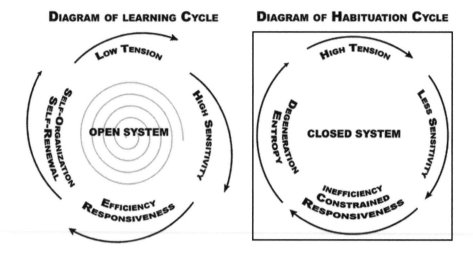

LOW TENSION

SELF-ORGANIZATION
SELF-RENEWAL

OPEN SYSTEM

HIGH SENSITIVITY

EFFICIENCY
RESPONSIVENESS

HIGH TENSION

DEGENERATION
ENTROPY

CLOSED SYSTEM

LESS SENSITIVITY

INEFFICIENCY
CONSTRAINED
RESPONSIVENESS

All living systems share a capacity for self-renewal. As conscious beings we can influence this process through awareness. Attention participates in the movement of regeneration, in the self-regulating and self-organizing of the whole. Theoretical physicist David Bohm describes the world of form as an abstraction from the indefinable and immeasurable movement of wholeness—the holomovement. Each abstraction unfolds from and enfolds into the whole, not as independent or separate parts but intrinsically related with all others, functioning as part of "all that is."

According to "consensual reality," the phenomena that make up our world are relatively fixed and independent, objects or entities existing over time. From this viewpoint, we see change as a process of modification, adding to or subtracting from an existing structure. Growth here has only limited meaning.

New possibilities emerge when we see ourselves and our world as the simultaneous enfolding and unfolding of form in the continuous movement of becoming, rather than as relatively fixed. Growth in this case represents a process of constant renewal.

Autopoiesis

Biologists Francisco Varela, Humberto Maturana, and Ricardo Uribe introduced the concept of "autopoiesis," the characteristic of living systems to continuously renew themselves and to regulate this process in such a way that the integrity of their structure is maintained. They write:

> Whereas a machine is geared to the output of a specific product, a biological cell is primarily concerned with renewing itself. Upgrading (anabolic) and downgrading (catabolic) processes run simultaneously. Not only the evolution of the system, but also its existence in a specific structure becomes dissolved into processes. In the domain of the living, there is little that is solid and rigid. An autopoetic structure results from the interaction of many processes.[2]

In complex organisms the capacity for regeneration arises from the ability of the intelligence of the whole to determine the functioning of the parts. A cell taken from an organism will live in a suitable culture for an extended period of time. However, it will eventually lose its differentiation, indicating that the whole determines the particular structure and functions of the individual cells.

The very ground substance that comprises our cells undergoes continuous transformation, disorganizing and reorganizing its structure and functions in a myriad of ways according to changing necessities. Research from the field of physiology illustrates this process. In his article "Structure and Properties of Ground Substances," James Oschman reports that studies have shown a structural and functional continuity of the matrix that comprises our cells' surroundings as well as its cytoplasmic and nucleic substance:

> We now recognize that the "structureless" cytoplasmic ground substance in fact contains various filaments, proteins, tubulin, actin, myosin, intermediate filaments, and microtubules. These are able to form as polymers, depolymerize, cross-link, intertwine, shape changes, cytoplasmic

streaming, pigment migrations, pinocytosis, secretion, mitosis, the myriad of activities that constitute life … The framework is a dynamic structure.…[3]

With awareness we can participate consciously in the process of self-renewal even at the level of our cells. When we differentiate our sensing of intrinsic movement, we become active participants in this self-organizing process through which we form. Rather than exploring a predetermined "reality" as an observer, we participate in the event, inventing and discovering simultaneously.

Some Soviet experiments demonstrated this in a simple way. Researchers found that

> … the eyes of the observer emit a force field that can influence what the eyes are looking at. These studies are performed by placing petri dishes containing yeast before persons with open eyes and before others with closed eyes and noting differences in the growth of the two sets of cultures. Open eyes increase yeast growth. More important, it is reported that the energy from the eyes is measurable and that some observers have a greater intensity of emission than others.[4]

A New Perspective on Healing, a New Way of Living

From the perspective of Somatic Learning, the process of healing necessitates change on the most fundamental level—in the very way we form ourselves soma-significantly.[5]

The term "soma-significating" emphasizes the one process that expresses itself physiologically and psychologically. This distinguishes it from the mechanical notion of "psychosomatic," which implies a causal relationship between parts and processes. From a psychosomatic standpoint, one might conclude that someone's cancer, asthma, or neck pain comes from repressed anger or the trauma of loss.

A fragmentary perspective tries to find relationships between separate parts. In a non- fragmentary, nondual perspective like Somatic Learning, we stop looking for relationships because we sense the intrinsic connectedness of the whole. In the above example, rather than thinking of the anger as causative, we see the physiological and psychological as different expressions of one process, the way we structure experience as a whole. In this sense, any situation can present an opportunity for inquiry as differentiating attention awakens a conscious participation in this self-organizing process.

For instance, the inquiry of an individual suffering from severe chronic pain illustrates how a problem that exists when we function in a fragmentary way may not even manifest when the organism functions integrally. Rather than trying to solve the "problem" of pain, we enter an inquiry that involves a change in the mode of experiencing.

A STUDENT'S FIRST EXPERIENCE

To give you some sense of how Somatic Learning can support someone in awakening somatic intelligence, I will share a description of one person's very first session. Though this account gives just a taste of what is possible, it represented a huge shift in Jerry's experience. Jerry suffered years of chronic pain and survived by doing the best he could to ignore his body. In this session, he began learning to be self-sensing and self-organizing, and the resulting diminishment of pain even in one session was enough to inspire him to begin a long journey. Jerry continued his study for years, and later trained to facilitate Somatic Learning with his own chronic-pain patients. This session was his first step along this journey of transformation.

Jerry, a practicing psychiatrist in his early sixties, had once been very active in sports, including running, cycling, and skiing. Over the years, however, he had become increasingly stiff, and simple activities such as sitting comfortably became virtually impossible. Jerry constantly struggled against gravity just to hold himself upright. A whiplash injury suffered in a car accident compounded his problems. His initial complaint was chronic neck and lower back pain, which severely restricted his mobility.

Jerry had sought relief from orthopedic surgeons, chiropractors, physical therapists, and acupuncturists, as well as exploring relaxation and visualization techniques to relieve the discomfort on his own—without success. When Jerry and I met for the first time, we didn't focus on his specific complaints, trying to cure or relieve his discomfort. Instead we began an inquiry into how he formed himself that brought about so much pain.

I began by asking Jerry to sense the way he sits. He had dropped into the chair, much like one might set down a sack of potatoes. As he spoke, I could see how much effort he mobilized just to sit there. He alternated between collapsing in on himself and rigidly tensing the muscles of the lower back, neck, and shoulders to hold himself erect.

When I asked him to sense into his sitting he began to observe his "body" with his "mind's eye" as if watching himself in a mirror. As Jerry focused, he exerted enormous effort to adjust his posture. He tried to compensate for his slouching, lifting himself by the neck and shoulders according to an image he held of correct posture. This took the pressure off his thoracic spine, but produced new stresses elsewhere in his structure.

I then asked Jerry to sit on a large gymnastic ball and experiment with slowly rolling the ball forward and back. As he began rolling the ball, his upper torso moved forward and backward, compensating for the change in his center of gravity. Then I provided some resistance that constrained any movement in space as he continued to roll the ball. Now Jerry could feel the support rise up from the ground through his spine like a wave. Eventually he could sense this omnidirectional wave extend and support his spine, whether he rolled the ball forward or back. He was no longer compensationally moving his "body like an object" in space. With his new level of differentiation, a subtle realm of intrinsic movement opened up that allowed him to "shape-shift." His structure self-organized in relation to the shifting center of gravity as he moved. As his spine extended, Jerry could sense the density of his upper back lighten and become less concretized.

Still the wave got caught in his neck. I asked him to notice how his visual perception was engaged in watching the movement in his "mind's eye." This constrained his eye movement, which held his head in a particular relationship to his torso while he observed his movement. I suggested that he close his eyes for a moment and sense the movement in his tissues, distinguishing between proprioception and visual perception. Once he could sense proprioceptively, I asked him to open his eyes. Soon he noticed that the wave no longer flowed freely through the top of his head but folded in on itself, creating some density in the upper back again. I suggested that Jerry once again close his eyes and visualize a horizon as far as he could see—then with his eyes still closed, to receive the horizon coming to him. Receiving the horizon in this way, Jerry could sense his head float almost like a bobble-head doll.

At this point, I asked Jerry to imagine himself opening his eyelids as though he were opening the shutters in an Italian villa to let the light in. I suggested it was possible to do so without tensing the eyes, without grasping to hold onto visual objects, but rather to let the light merely flow through his head as if through an empty room, its radiance pouring through a window at the back of his skull into the gardens beyond. Then I asked him to open his eyes, as though he were opening the shutters, allowing his eyes to rest like buoys upon the horizon floating toward the back of his head. Now Jerry could see in a new way, allowing his visual perception to take in his surroundings, including me, without his eyes becoming fixated. At this point, his visual perception and proprioception functioned independently. Not only did this free his head, it enabled him to sustain the somatic meditation while his eyes were open and actively perceiving the world around him.

Once he had differentiated clearly the vertical axis of the wave, he sensed the extension of his spine from the base through the top of his head. Now I invited Jerry to extend his presence along the horizontal axis. As the wave rose through his thoracic spine, I asked Jerry to sense a "hair's breadth of space" between his shoulder blades and his back (almost as though someone had blown through a straw into this narrow space). This floated his shoulders. Then I asked him to extend his presence all at once, through the whole length of his arms, from what I like to refer to as "the medial edge of the wing tip" (at the scapula) to the lateral edge (in the fingertips.) Now he could catch this updraft of wind through the whole length of his "wings" from tip to tip. Once the weight of his shoulder girdle was no longer hanging like a yoke around his neck, he felt no more pain or chronic constriction in his neck.

Then I encouraged Jerry to consider the possibility of coming to standing without lifting himself up. I suggested that he could, instead, pour his weight into the ground like grains pouring through a silo, and allow gravity to support him. I recommended that he stand by anchoring his sacrum as he straightened his knees. He was surprised to find that he could stand without tensing his surface skeletal muscles. The sensation of floating upright was pleasurable to him. As we began to move through space, he commented on how different he felt—more grounded and lighter. The pains in his knees and spine were all gone. As I conducted his sensing to receive the ground rising up through him, he took delight in discovering greater vitality and ease in his structure.

We then translated the experience he had on the ball to sitting on a stool. Now while rolling an imaginary ball, he sensed the wave arising through his spine. I began to facilitate his self-sensing and self-organizing once again by offering resistance—holding him at the front, between the two bones of his shins, while he rolled the invisible ball forward. And then at the back of his shins while he rolled the ball away from me. Gradually I offered less and less support through my touch as he replaced my touch with the touch of an invisible partner. I suggested that he enjoy receiving the support of the touch moving through and beyond his structure at the same time that he "kissed backed," sensing the interpenetration flowing in all directions.

I invited Jerry to practice speaking while still sensing, giving voice to what he was feeling without disengaging from his somatic awareness to talk "about" it. In this way, Jerry began to integrate his emotional and cognitive intelligence with his somatic intelligence. Every once in a while, he would catch himself working to communicate something and noticed that he was no longer actively sensing. We labeled that "efforting." I suggested that each time he caught himself "efforting," he could simply stop "rowing upstream" and sense what happens. Inevitably, as soon as the efforting stopped, he felt relief. And once again, riding the waves of joy and interest, he felt renewed.

Through this self-sensing and self-organizing process, Jerry learned how to see, sit, stand, walk, and talk in a new way, dramatically reducing the chronic tension and pain in the lower back and neck that he had found crippling at times.

In moving, Jerry began to sense the way he responded to the ground. The movement awakened awareness in a similar way that we may notice a grasshopper as it leaps about but fail to notice it standing quite still on the lawn. Rather than moving to cultivate strength or to stretch, Jerry began to differentiate his awareness to the subtle changes that occur continuously even when sitting or standing motionless. At this point in the experiment, Jerry had distinguished between watching himself, which occurs in linear time (time flowing from the past toward the future), and sensing that occurs in the present. In the fragmentation of watching ourselves, we either anticipate the movement, controlling it through thought like a choreographer directing a dance, or we follow the movement, watching it like a scientist observes phenomena. In either case we dissociate by getting ahead of or following behind the actual process of moving. And from the "here" of our stationary "control tower" in the head, we watch something moving "there"—as in the pelvis.

When Jerry felt the difference between watching from a point outside the movement and sensing from within, his breathing deepened considerably. Not needing to hold his neck still in order to watch, his head and torso now moved with greater ease, supported from below as he received the forces rising from the ground through his pelvis and lengthening his spine.

In sensing, Jerry differentiated the process of sitting in such a way that it now involved an active responsiveness to the gravitational field. As he relaxed the habitual tensing of the surface skeletal muscles, he received the support of the "ground" rising up through each vertebra and buoying his head. Jerry felt suspended vertically. His spine elongated like a wave spiraling upward with each breath. He found that even when he no longer actively moved in space, he moved intrinsically, his structure responding to the ground as he breathed.

A radical change had occurred. Jerry did not merely manage his pain differently or adjust his posture. He no longer had the problem to "work" on. Jerry's old, fragmentary way of forming experience no longer interfered with the organism's ability to self-organize.

Implications

The implications of this work go far beyond repair, relief of pain, and return of lost functioning. The traditional medical concept of recovery, or even healing, no longer seems adequate. Perhaps "wholing" better describes this change from a fragmentary mode of functioning into a mode of living from a more awakened somatic intelligence that is self-sensing, self-organizing, and self-renewing.

As a child, I watched a show on television where people sent in little lines on a piece of paper and out of these squiggles an artist rendered a drawing of whatever it was in the sender's imagination. I was very impressed with his ability to draw something specific (maybe a clown, a lake with ducks, or a horse) that someone had requested from these random notations. It was obvious that the artist very much enjoyed the challenge of connecting all the dots and dashes. It is like that for me when

I begin the exploration of Somatic Learning with a new student. I like to inquire about how their deepest longing lives in them (what they yearn for most), as well as what concerns and challenges them.

The session is designed according to the inquiry, in relation to what is most meaningful in the person's life at present. With newly differentiated attention, they notice as straining occurs and learn how to relax out of the straining, as opposed to compensating for it. In this way they open into greater freedom and aliveness by receiving the unbounded spaciousness and surrendering into the free fall. They learn to extend their presence into the space this creates in their experience. It's a subtle shift in awareness that opens the space in which to extend … and it only needs to be a hair's breadth of space. Once you learn to invent and discover space within, you can keep opening infinitely. We are not trying to connect the dots of meaning, but begin holding the field of meaning broad enough for everything to light up as a whole, like the blanket of stars in the midnight sky.

The name I gave to the Institute of Somatic Learning is "Inquiry" because I think about entering into any practice as entering into an inquiry. The inquiry continues to reward you at whatever depth of subtlety you are willing to engage your attention. The implicate order continues to open the more you deepen your feeling, sensing, knowing—expanding your presence into the unknown. The unknown becomes intimate with you through shared presence as the inquiry continues opening. I think of the longings, concerns, and challenges as forces of necessity and opportunity that call us into deepening the inquiry. We can use the circumstances and conditions that arise in life as opportunities to receive the infinite and to participate creatively and compassionately with all that is.

Unlike many therapeutic modalities, Somatic Learning does not have a prescribed technology or set routine that is one-size-fits-all. The client does not come in and go through a package or predetermined series. The facilitator takes up whatever is most alive and immediate. In this way, effort is not necessary to induce change. Like a plant, the structure grows out of its yearning for the light, without any secondary act of will.

MORE FIRST-TIME EXPERIENCES

Following are short descriptions by students after their first encounter with Somatic Learning.

"The most amazing thing about Somatic Learning is that my own body has retrained itself! When I awoke in the morning and got out of bed, my body had taken on an entirely new alignment—'spine in front, horizon behind me.' I went for a hike, and everything was different: my back was released from strain, and my body was realigned along a much healthier axis. On the hike, everything felt easier. A week later, my body is still holding this new alignment effortlessly. I remind myself all the time: spine in front, horizon in back. Everything is functioning better thanks to this profoundly simple work, and I look forward to going deeper."—*Steve Bhaerman*

From a woman a month after giving birth:

"I cannot tell you in words how thankful I am for the Somatic Learning work. I am clear that the elongations I practiced contributed to my speedy and unusual cervical ripening. Also, my husband and I are amazed by the work with our little boy (four weeks old). He is breathing more calmly, sleeping a lot more, crying only for short periods of time, and not as desperately."—*Gitta Sivander*

From a woman coming in with intense pain from a bulging disc:

"I just wanted to tell you again how much of a miracle I think this whole process has been, and how grateful I am for your incredible wisdom and help at this most crucial moment. I am changing my life/DNA/ thoughts, and now am really following my spirit. To think that I went from considering a cortisone injection two days ago to this kind of grounded mobility—that's huge."—*Katayoon Zand Zakili*

"The experience of my first session of Somatic Learning was life-changing. I feel changes on the physical, mental, emotional, and spiritual level. Old pains disappeared. Plus, I released myself from the bondage of a two-year mentally and emotionally debilitating situation by forgiving myself as well as the other person involved. I feel that my core 'antenna' connection has been rewired so that I easily feel that I am in the flow and grounded. All of this happened within the first four days. And even better is the realization that I am aware and in command of the process of realigning myself, moment by moment. The practice is masterful in conveying the experience of somatic intelligence with love, kindness, and compassion. What a Blessing—all the way around."—*Trudy Siewert Bhaerman*

The Somatic Meditations are not intended to improve or fix problems or conditions of the past, but arise out of a deep acceptance and appreciation of what is … *the embrace* as described in Chapter 4. When we learn to receive "what is" as a gift … we are poised to participate creatively in how we are forming ourselves and our world, in the here and now. This is a practice of self-mastery … lucidly awakening as the dreamer, dreaming the dream into appearance. Self-mastery is the process of finding and losing and finding awareness again, each time we fall back asleep. Like setting up an experiment to see light reflected as a wave rather than a particle, our practice sets up the experiment of living to awaken in each moment to the luminous consciousness that we are.

The whole concept of "fixing the body" seems so presumptuous, since somatic intelligence is a far more pervasive and subtle intelligence than the "thought" attempting to fix it. Somatic intelligence awakens ever-greater freedom and aliveness in the process of transformative learning and change. In the practice, the problems that arose at more limited dimensions of consciousness resolve themselves organically, just as an apparent paradox can resolve itself from a higher-dimensional perspective.

Somatic Meditations

Somatic Meditations are designed to support you in dimensionally extending your presence, down the rabbit hole, into a wonderland of possibility.

Many problems that existed in your prior habitual state will no longer exist. Some will reappear from time to time, when something triggers old programming. As you integrate the practice, your sensing will become more differentiated. You will begin to sense and respond to increasingly subtle change and movement.

> I do not view post-traumatic stress disorder as a pathology to be managed, suppressed, or adjusted to, but the result of a natural process gone awry. Healing trauma requires a direct experience of the living, feeling, knowing organism.
> —*Peter Levine, PhD*[6]

Your somatic intelligence will be able to integrate functions that previously operated mechanically from early programming and trauma (or compensations for them). As this intelligence matures, you develop a more subtle "energy body" capable of many things that the "object body" could not do—self-organizing and self-renewing in a way that transforms both structure and functioning, which continues to support more learning. You become pervasively learning-oriented, functioning much more efficiently and gracefully. This flowering of our somatic intelligence can become a new referent for aging as a process of maturing gracefully.

> Because such reactions to constant stress can build up over sustained periods of time, the resultant chronic muscular contractions are associated with aging. But age is not a causative factor. Time, in itself, is neutral. It is what happens during our lifetime that causes muscular reflexes to habituate. Accumulated stress and trauma are the causes of sensory-motor amnesia, and what we mistakenly ascribe to the effects of "old age" are the direct effects of sensory-motor amnesia.
>
> There is no bodily "cure" for sensory-motor amnesia. The chronic muscular rigidities habituated during aging are impervious to medical remedies. Third-person manipulations are of no avail.
>
> There is, however, a way of releasing the involuntary restrictions of

sensory-motor amnesia: it is somatic learning. If one focuses one's awareness on an unconscious, forgotten area of the soma, one can begin to perceive a minimal sensation that is just sufficient to direct a minimal movement, and this, in turn, gives new sensory feedback of that area which, again, gives a new clarity of movement, etc.

This sensory feedback associates with adjacent sensory neurons, further clarifying the synergy that is possible with the associated motor neurons. This makes the next motor effort inclusive of a wider range of associated voluntary neurons, thus broadening and enhancing the motor action and, thereby, further enhancing the sensory feedback. This back-and-forth motor procedure gradually "wedges" the amnesiac area back into the range of volitional control: the unknown becomes known and the forgotten becomes relearned.

A soma that is maximally free is a soma that has achieved a maximal degree of voluntary control and a minimal degree of involuntary conditioning. This state of autonomy is an optimal state of individuation, i.e., one having a highly differentiated repertoire of response possibilities to environmental stimuli.

The state of somatic freedom is, in many senses, the optimal human state. Looked at from a third-person, bodily viewpoint, somatic freedom is a state of maximal efficiency and minimal entropy.

—*Thomas Hanna*[7]

Transforming Your Relationship to Gravity and Aging

A major benefit of Somatic Learning is that it helps you transform your relationship to two things that have been seen as unalterably fixed: gravity and aging.

To make such a claim sounds like magic. But if it is, it's not the kind of magic that depends on medications, injections, and surgery, or any remedy directed "from the outside in," from an image/object orientation. As you will discover for yourself when you read this book and practice Somatic Learning in your own life, every amazing result comes from within. Somatic intelligence will transform your relationship to gravity and aging—and much, much more.

Why gravity and aging? What's the connection? Attributing many of the problems of aging and pain to time and gravity seems simplistic at best. I see both time and gravity as neutral forces. For instance, research in healthy people has shown no significant loss of brain tissue even in people in their ninth decade. The cortical thinning or loss of brain tissue is not correlated to time itself. Likewise, the common problems of structural deterioration associated with gravity and aging arise not from gravity itself, but from our adversarial relationship to gravity. While this book is not about overcoming the effects of gravity, it does open up a valuable inquiry into how we can invent and discover a new reality by partnering with gravity. Not only can we let go of the burden of gravity as "a negative pull downward," but gravity can actually deliver us from habitual patterns that have become concretized in our structure and functioning. The learning and change we undergo in the process of healing transforms every aspect of our living. This work offers more than simply relief from strain and pain: it serves as a portal into the process of self-renewal.

Partnering with Gravity Will Lead You to a New Reality

Transforming your relationship to gravity transforms how you age. In the Somatic Meditations, gravity serves as the feedback enabling us to see which course our lives are taking—learning and self-renewal or habituation and degeneration … And we see this now rather than at the tail end of life when it is too late to make a difference. If you have an adversarial relationship to gravity, if you are "fighting" or struggling to "overcome" gravity, your aging will be characterized by degeneration and entropy.[8]

Transforming your relationship to gravity provides the real-time feedback you need to sustain a learning orientation that is self-sensing, self-organizing, and self-renewing. When you enjoy a creative partnership with gravity, you receive the support that rises when the ground breaks your fall toward the center of the earth. You feel your connection to all that is. You move effortlessly from a fluid responsiveness. From this alliance with gravity, you will evolve through the years with wisdom, grace, and gratefulness. As you grow in years, you can experience ever-greater freedom and aliveness. Your "aging" becomes negentropic.

> Another long-term consequence of meditation is that there is less cortical thinning with aging. That is most pronounced in the anterior cingulate cortex, that area we were talking about involving the integration of feeling and thinking. There are some suggestive findings that some form of contemplative or religious practice can reduce the cognitive declines normally associated with aging, such as what occurs in extreme conditions like Alzheimer's disease.
> —*Drs. Rick Hanson and Richard Mendius*[9]

Either entropy or evolution will prevail. From the old paradigm, we appear like helpless subjects of evolution—from the perspective of Somatic Learning, we are evolution. Seeing that our lives are at stake fans the fire of attention.

Steve's Story: Letting Go of Efforting

A fifty-year-old man named Steve Star, working as a chef and organic farmer, injured his neck in a tractor accident. His practice of Somatic Learning softened him, revealing tender beauty that had previously been masked by all of his straining and efforting "to be enough."

When I first hurt my neck I followed the time-honored male tradition of ignoring the pain. As stiffness set in over the next couple of months I would pop my neck to release the stiffness. This spiraled downward, to more stiffness and pain, until I finally decided I needed some help and went to a chiropractor.

My first visit to the chiropractor involved a full spinal X-ray. While looking at the X-ray I could clearly see the developing bone spurs between C6 and C7. However, I also noticed cloudiness around three mid-thoracic vertebrae. When I asked him about it he simply shrugged it off as calcification that was a normal part of the aging process. I was somewhat shocked by his answer; I felt there must be some way to address this problem. This motivated me to look for an alternative solution.

I had been to a Somatic Learning workshop in which Dr. Kaparo treated a young woman with neurofibromatosis. I was standing behind her when she demonstrated one of the Somatic Meditations she called "riding the wave of the breath." I was astonished as I saw this wave of movement ripple up her spine. I remember thinking: I want to do that too. After three sessions of Somatic Learning the pain was gone, and I felt empowered, because I was now confident I could maintain my own health.

But what was happening did not fit any model or experience that I previously had. I was trying to understand what was going on, having come from a scientific background. I had a degree in biology and statistics. I expected things to be logical. The practice clearly worked, though I could not imagine why. I had never experienced my body at such subtle levels before.

I remember that a couple of months into the practice, I got up in the middle of the night and started doing some elongations in the dark (remembering Dr. Kaparo's story of playing blindfolded). It was the first time I experienced a wave go up my spine, and suddenly I started to get it. The irony was that the first time I really felt the wave, I had made the conscious decision to do a standing elongation, going through the steps of it, but at some point my mind drifted away. And then I suddenly noticed a wave go through my structure without really having made the effort to make it happen. I realized in that moment that efforting didn't work, but I was so programmed to believe that nothing happened without effort that I efforted anyway.

Disenthralling myself from the pattern of "efforting" has been the main focus of my practice. For instance, even after several years of practice, I still find the snake breathing very useful because I can hear how I use my breath to effort. Any straining shows up as an irregularity in the flow of the exhale, disrupting the smooth sound. Often I realize I've missed the opportunity to relax at all. I pass through the inhale in my rush to the next exhale, so I can keep "working it" rather than resting into a pose and enjoying it. When I do that, I end up forcing the exhale. To use the surfing analogy, I'm staying in front of the wave paddling my head off rather than riding it.

When asked what compelled him to teach Somatic Learning, Steve describes the satisfaction he feels from empowering others to change their situation.

It's like the old adage about the difference between giving a man a fish for dinner and teaching him how to fish. When I can support other people in a way that I know empowers them for the rest of their lives rather than making them comfortable temporarily, I feel satisfied in the work I'm doing.

My wife also experienced dramatic results from Somatic Learning after tearing her rotator cuff. She had been doing what the doctor and the physical therapist said, but when she started practicing Somatic Meditations, she experienced what a difference her own inner awareness made. It's not that she was unwilling to take responsibility for her body, or unwilling to do the work. But the information she was given came from the same perspective from which the problem originally arose, and so never quite addressed the problem itself. Treating the symptoms rather than the cause kept falling short of full healing and led to a sense of failure and frustration. Becoming self-sensing and self-organizing, she began to live in her body differently. From the feedback she got from the sensations in her shoulders, she learned to move her arms without straining. This was her breakthrough.

A human being is a part of a whole, called by us universe, a part limited in time and space. He experiences himself, his thoughts and feelings, as something separated from the rest … a kind of optical delusion of his consciousness. This delusion is a kind of prison for us, restricting us to our personal desires and to affection for a few persons nearest to us. Our task must be to free ourselves from this prison by widening our circle of compassion to embrace all living creatures and the whole of nature in its beauty.

—*Albert Einstein*[1]

CHAPTER 4

The Embrace

The primary intention behind Somatic Learning practice goes beyond healing the body. The body will heal and renew itself as soon as we get out of the way … when we stop straining and compensating. We must stop perpetuating the violence of living in fragmentation, identifying with an image that separates us from our direct experiencing. The primary intention of the art and practice of Somatic Learning is *awakening*.

The body provides us with the perfect learning environment for breaking our identification with the image/object reality. It enables awakening to who we truly are as infinite consciousness. Through its finely tuned feedback system we can sense the difference between functioning as an object moving through space and our presencing of spaciousness, fluidly unfolding as movement within movement. We are generally unaware of the incoherencies inherent in our system of thought, since thought does not recognize itself as a participant in what it sees. What a Somatic Learning practice can provide is a context for sensing how the mind is forming us in each moment.

It is relatively easy to produce what is referred to as a "state-specific effect." Many therapeutic modalities can achieve effects that are only temporary, dependent on a mode of functioning that is not sustainable. We find evidence of this phenomenon in research on healing and multiple personality disorder. Even in this context, extraordinary adaptive responses to extremity have been documented.

> You needn't heal your wounds.
> They can fade as stars from the morning sky.
> Consider how in a severely traumatized person,
> scars sometimes disappear instantly
> with the shift from one to another of multiple personalities.
> Burns left by parents extinguishing their cigarettes into a baby's flesh,
> even these disappear.
> Diabetes, high blood pressure, allergies, come and go.
> The only reason you think yourself continuous
> is that every time you check,
> you're there.
> —*Risa Kaparo from "The Invocation"*[2]

Through the practice of Somatic Learning you can gain or improve your innate ability to facilitate a shift in consciousness and organismic functioning that can manifest a different reality immediately, even when chronic problems have persisted. However, this change generally does not sustain itself, and many people reexperience the problems that presented in their previous state.

For this reason, I have devoted my exploration and research to the possibility of realizing a different generalized order … as it didn't interest me to relieve someone's pain, for instance, if it was just going to keep manifesting. I had no interest in growing a person's dependence on me to provide relief. I am interested in what changes the order in a sustainable way. I am committed to developing and teaching practices that provide a context for transformative learning, healing, and change that is self-sustaining.

The Somatic Learning practices are non-coercive and non-interventionist. Rather than fixing the "body," they arise from the intention of receiving the gift of "what is" through embodiment. Coming to know ourselves through an awakened somatic intelligence dispels the habits of fragmentation that are the "curse" of this stage of our evolution.

Fable

To bring this point home, I will share a fairy tale that expresses this challenge metaphorically. Do you remember the old Arthurian tale in which the knight of most impeccable integrity, Sir Gawain, agrees to marry the grotesque old hag, Lady Ragnell, for she alone possesses the power to save the King?

Our story begins far back in the eighth century when the woods were full and the sky clear, and the young King Arthur went out with his royal entourage to hunt. The path was long and winding, the chase hard, and soon Arthur, the swiftest of them all, became separated from his men. He found himself alone with only a bow and arrow for defense, lost among tall trees and deep ferns, the deer path hidden in the thick underbrush. But the king was not really alone; unbeknownst to him, he had been watched.

"You are Arthur," said a large man with weapons. "I am Sir Grommer, and I will kill you for your trespass on my sacred lands." The young king shook and trembled with unaccustomed fright. Grommer began to smile. "I see that you are weak, all alone; maybe I have been too harsh. I will give you one chance for life. Take it or die. I have a riddle for you. If you can tell me what women most desire"—he laughed outright with a sneer playing around the corners of his mouth—"I will spare you. I give you one year to find the one true answer." Grommer left after marking the place and time of their next fateful meeting. Arthur made his way slowly, head hanging low, through the woods to return to his men, his horse, and his castle.

"What is troubling you, Sir?" asked Gawain, the bravest and wisest of all the king's knights.

"My fate, and the fate of this kingdom, is hanging on a riddle," said Arthur, and he told Gawain the riddle. Arthur spoke to Gawain, his voice for the first time showing a hint of fear. "This realm's fate hangs on a single thread. Solve this or all will be lost."

"We will find the answer," said Gawain. "Someone in this great land will know. So the two searched for a year, far and wide, low and high, asking maidens and milkmaids, wise men, wizards, and old women— many women, for it was their words they trusted most. They collected twelve bound volumes of answers, but to no avail, none had the ring of truth. And so a year passed; Grommer's day was drawing near. Arthur rode out alone deep in thought, for he had nothing to give and his life seemed forfeit for lack of the true answer. The noonday sun was hot. Soon Arthur grew drowsy, and sought rest under the leaves of an ancient oak tree. Through half-shut eyes he saw a hideous hag whose form was like no other. This woman loomed large and wide, with wild and greasy hair. From her body the raw stench of rotting bone nauseated all who drew near. He rubbed his eyes in disbelief, but she was still there.

"You are Arthur the cursed king who will soon die," she said revealing rotten teeth and stale breath. "I am the Lady Ragnell, the one who holds the answer that will surely save your life," she cackled with a hideous grin.

"In twelve months time I have found many answers," said Arthur. "Be gone old woman!"

"Your answers hold no truth," she said with a confidence that caused the king to ply her with offers of bags of gold, jewels, kingdoms, castles....

"Tell me, tell me, and a king's ransom shall be yours."

"What need do I have for all your riches," she spat with a terrible grin. In all your vast kingdom there is nothing I crave. There is only one thing I desire," said Lady Ragnell. "Sir Gawain, your wisest knight must become my husband."

"No, he is not mine to offer."

"I ask not that you give him to me, only that you beseech him if he will, and if he agrees I will answer your riddle. If not, you will die." The thought of that most noble knight marrying the wretch was impossible, but not as impossible as his fateful meeting with Sir Grommer. Arthur could not help but ask Gawain, and though the king pleaded against it, telling him of the hag's hideous visage, Gawain was determined to make the sacrifice.

"It is an honor, my King, that I can marry and save your life."

So the witch whispered her secret, and two days later, Arthur appeared before Grommer. Hoping to spare Gawain from his terrible fate, Arthur opened the first of the twelve volumes and read off each answer, one by one and each was denied. As the night wore on, Grommer sharpened his sword for the king's death drew nigh, and at the final moment just before the first crack of daylight, he came at last to the words he dreaded most: the witch's answer. "It seems," he said, "that what women want is only one thing: Sovereignty."

These words released the king from his vow. Arthur's life was saved. Arthur begged Gawain to postpone the day of the wedding, on the grounds that marriage was no longer necessary. He was free, and the kingdom saved. But the knight—honorable and true—was determined to keep his word.

Throughout the grand wedding feast Gawain attended kindly to the needs of his new wife, though all turned away from her wretched face and the court whispered about the strange marriage.

After the couple withdrew to their chambers for the dreaded marriage night, Lady Ragnell spoke thus to her husband. "You have kept your vows well, but do you not owe me something? Come now and kiss me, my husband."

At the touch of her lips, Gawain was astonished to find that he was kissing a fair young maiden.

"I've surprised you, have I not?" she said, twirling round before his admiring gaze. "Do you prefer me in this form?" she said with a half smile. "Sir Grommer always hated me for my quick will. He cast a spell which with your kiss you have partway broken. But now I ask, do you want me this way in the court or in the bedchamber, for I can only be beautiful for half the day. What will you choose, my knight?"

Gawain looked at the lovely form and remembered the hag with her rotting bones and terrible stench. He paused, thinking, in silence, then stated, "This is not a choice I can make. It is your choice, my dearest. Fair by day, fair by night, whatever your choice I will abide you." At these words the curse was completely dispelled and Ragnell came into full bloom. So began the lives of Sir Gawain and his Lady.

After the couple withdraw from the wedding feast to their bedchambers, when Lady Ragnell says to her husband, "You have kept your vows well … come now and kiss me, my husband," surely Gawain must have had to extend past all the reactions the old hag triggered for him, the dismay and revulsion, to kiss the hideous creature that stood before him. After all, she was said to bear the most foul odor and have hair growing from the moles on her huge hooked nose, and she drooled between the few remaining teeth that rotted away in her mouth.

In the realm of myth and fairytale, the characters in the story are archetypes, representing different aspects of the psyche. The knight is the animus, the inner masculine or yang force of light, and the old hag represents the shadow side of the inner feminine aspect. In her abandoned state she is grotesque. Unable to flow freely, passion and vital energy are locked within this rejected aspect of the self. She is dried up. Old.

In the archetypal realm, we often encounter the leitmotif of an embrace transfiguring what was previously identified as old and ugly into a youthful beauty. This is the soul-engendering embrace.

When the old hag is received into the folds of the self—her beauty and innocence is revealed, she is renewed. However, she cannot stay like this. The old scripts reassert themselves, and she falls into the gravity pull of her habitual response patterns. In the words of Silvan Tomkins, "The world we perceive is a dream we learn to have from a script we have not written."[3]

> "Do you prefer me in this form?" she said with a half smile. "Sir Grommer always hated me for my quick will. He cast a spell which with your kiss you have partway broken. But now I ask, do you want me this way in the court or in the bedchamber, for I can only be beautiful for half the day. What will you choose, my knight?" Gawain looked at the lovely form and remembered the hag. He paused, thinking, in silence …

As long as we live in the duality of private and public worlds, of inside and outside, the fragmentation can never resolve itself, thus the second half of the curse. We remain enthralled by images, memory. How can we stand in a room full of mirrors and not identify with the images reflected back? Breaking the spell of how we know ourselves inferentially, we disenthrall ourselves from the identification with images, which is the curse we live under.

The deeper integration is the real challenge to all of us who have been moved by such a transformative experience. In my own journey, as I believe in many, the wounds of childhood opened me to forces beyond imagination. And still, I kept falling flat on my face. Unable to sustain the passion of Eros in my life, I saw mirrored to me the ways I felt not enough. It showed me how dependent I was on an externally reflected sense of self to avert the chronic shame echoing through my life. Confronted with a life-threatening illness, I was sent through another portal on the journey, and again with some initiations by fire: the trials of loss, and motherhood. I entered each learning to embrace what is.

In what areas have you found your life wanting? Calling you forth?

When we are thankful for some experiences and not others, picking and choosing, we miss the grace in each moment, the opportunity. When we take up "what is" with gratefulness, our shame is transformed into humility and awe.

"It is a choice I cannot make, dear Lady Ragnell. It concerns you. Fair by day, fair by night, whatever your choice I will abide you." At these words the curse was completely dispelled....

The fairytale takes us to the necessity of meeting what arises—not processing it through aversion and attraction, grasping after what we want or avoiding what we don't want, but to the embrace of what is.[4] In the embrace our inherent beauty and intelligence are revealed to us. The first half of the curse is dispelled—the curse of fragmentation. This part of the curse can often be dispelled in a single moment. This is not a rare occurrence. In fact, I experience it with people in each session and workshop. We've all met such pregnant moments—where somehow we've been able to receive ourselves—without valuing this over that, without moving away from or toward something else. Where we take up what is here and now, and suddenly everything feels equally dispersed, weightless, flowing freely. What appears on the surface—what we're becoming—is at once reconciled with the depths of our innate intelligence. In that space there is always innocence and awe. And beauty. And the truest expression of gratitude—which is fruitfulness, renewal, giving birth to oneself.

> "Wife" is the optimal term that may be applied to the soul. It is even above "virgin." That within himself, a man should receive god is good: and, receiving god, the man is still virgin. Nevertheless, it is better that god should be fruitful through him, for fruitfulness alone is real gratitude for god's gift, and in fruitfulness the soul is a wife, with newborn gratitude....
> —*Meister Eckhart*[5]

The difficulty is that when this somatic insight hits us, it is usually not sustainable. Something happens that triggers the old scripts, and suddenly we find ourselves an old hag or an ugly monster again, whether in the court or the bedchamber. Even though we now know there is another realm of possibility equally real and coexisting with this one, somehow we keep returning to the old order. And so the process by which we come into a new order represents another challenge in the learning cycle. Being new, "virgin," and beginning in beauty is a double necessity that is only initiated with an unconditional embrace of what is.

Krishnamurti often posed the question of how to live in the world and not of it. We must learn to live in a way not defined by the old order, or preexisting self-construct.

We make real the private world or public space by the movement of attention without seeing the source, the minding process that is holding it, focusing on it, creating it. When the minding process itself lights up we see both the public and private worlds as two reflections of the movement of consciousness, and suddenly we stop going back and forth.

The back-and-forth movement of attention gives way to a new mode of sensing the movement of wholeness, as it lights up from the inside out—without focusing from anywhere.

When this happens, the duality of private world and public space— the bedchamber and the court—disappears. The dichotomy resolves itself without any act of will. It's not that we learn to deal with it—the resolution of that conflict between private world and public space occurs when the field of awareness becomes dimensionally extended so that both the bedchamber and the court are seen and experienced as one movement—a higher-dimensional reality.

We change the ground of reality though our participation, inventing and discovering a whole that opens infinitely, renewing itself. Rather than choosing between worlds—giving value to this over that—to function in either world, we live in the space where the two worlds meet. Here we no longer have to choose. We awaken to greater freedom—awareness without fragmentation.

For some, self-consciousness is the curse that afflicts more pervasively when they are in public space. For others, the fear of being alone, rejected, or abandoned, etc., can trigger old shame scripts that turn us back into the old hag. Sometimes someone may be moving easily through life and suddenly he or she gets sucked into a psycho-bio-energetic black hole paralyzed by shame. Because of the self-perpetuating nature of shame scripts, the affect "shame" (a biological reaction), instead of becoming conscious as feeling, turns into emotion when biographized by our self-talk. As we become more identified with the stories we tell ourselves, emotion turns into a perpetual mood or state … like depression.[6]

> The breeze at dawn has secrets to tell you.
> Don't go back to sleep!
> You must ask for what you really want.
> Don't go back to sleep!
> People are going back and forth across the doorsill
> where the two worlds touch. The Door is round and open.
> Don't go back to sleep!
>   —*Jalaluddin Rumi*[7]

Dispelling the whole curse means not going back to sleep. The challenge of the second half of the curse is this: to take up each moment as the gift of opportunity to receive the whole—now, and now, and now. You must not fall asleep to what your deepest love wants if the embrace is to become a new order. I cannot hold on to an insight without losing its beauty and newness. The insight itself must become self-sustaining in each moment. This is the challenge of ongoing practice in the art of awakening.

All the habitual tension, the strain patterns, the pain we experience living in the field of gravity are like the moles growing on Lady Ragnell's face and the decaying of her teeth and her bad breath and sour smell. What happens when we listen through all that and find the ground that sustains us, that is the first embrace. An inversion occurs when everything we have done to compensate for bearing this burden begins to unravel itself. We find that what we had experienced as a burden (like gravity) has now delivered us from all our strain. No secondary act of will is necessary.

I see people in workshops come into a way of moving like upright water and then, when I call for a break, they suddenly move their object body around with all the same constraints that they had before. Though they do not have those same physical constraints anymore, they reconstruct them because that is who they think they are. Their image/identity has all these constraints built into it.

So now the challenge of getting from where you are sitting to the water fountain is learning to receive the ground moving through you, to sense gravity drawing you to the center of the earth, the ground breaking your fall, the force rising up from the earth, space moving through you. There is a nonsequential aspect to the movement like an electron jumping from one orbit to another without having gone through the space in between. You are unfolding as form and enfolding back into the undifferentiated wholeness, simultaneously. Rather than a continuity of self that is moving through time and space, we can become awake to how the whole renews itself in this moment through our movement.

Note the difference between Lady Ragnell going about her business in the court and bedchamber in a split or divided sense of self, and this fresh unfolding presence participating in connection to all that is (as a continuity of form). This nondual awareness is self-sensing, self-organizing, and self-renewing.

Sovereignty

When we interpret the story of Sir Gawain and Lady Ragnell archetypally, we explore the relationship of the animus to the anima.

One might think that what women really want is to be loved fully, but what does that mean? In the story, the masculine (the animus) aspect of our human experience will often relate to the feminine according to the masculine value of perfection. Within this value system, the feminine will feel inadequate, deficient, ugly, and will tend toward an incessant attempt to improve herself, trying to be worthy or pleasing, or giving up when the burden of shame becomes unbearable, hardening in self-contempt. In the extreme, we see this problem expressed as eating disorders as well as addictive and obsessive behavior patterns.

The way that the feminine in each of us longs to be loved is in her sovereignty, to be taken up, received and given forth, renewed, on the edge of her becoming. When she is aligned with her deepest somatic intelligence, riding the waves of her joy and interest, she feels loved and accepted as she is, here and now.

Sovereignty implies freedom. But what is freedom? We tend to think of freedom as choice. When we are feeling ambivalent or torn between one desire that lives in conflict with another, we have to ignore certain needs and feelings and impulses to go with others. In contrast, when we extend our presence to take up the whole movement of feeling within us from a new depth, the paradox—or what appears an inherent opposition between these different necessities—resolves itself. We come to a soft landing with a greater extension of presence where the surface of our behavior and thoughts is congruent with the depths of our feeling/sensing/knowing. We are made whole and function from a new coherence. In this way, we redefine freedom as obedience from the etymological roots of the word: to listen thoroughly. Krishnamurti referred to this as "choice-less awareness."

Sovereignty in this sense refers to the loving embrace of what is, beyond values and images, attractions and aversions, dispelling the curse of the fragmentation, dissociation, separation, and inner conflict.

> … anything or anyone
> that does not bring you alive
> you have made too small for you.
> —*David Whyte*

At times, when we meet someone, where the dimensional extension of their presence resonates with the dimensional extension of ours, and we feel taken up and received and synergistically given forth, renewed, we are held in this magnetic field of the co-resonance. This is the embrace.

Most of the time we diminish ourselves to fit with the images reflected to us as children, when we were seen not for who we are, but how we fit our parents' needs and aversions.

As children, we were completely dependent on our parents for all the sustenance we needed to grow. In order to sustain connection with our

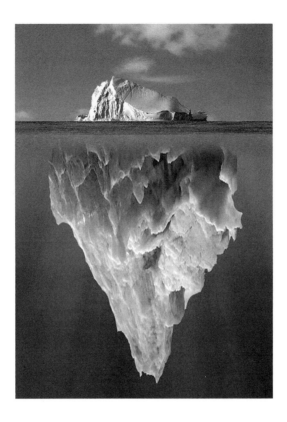

parents we gave value to the image they projected on us, carrying forth the hope of belonging. However, often the image was incongruent with the depth of our experiencing. This incongruence leaves us feeling insecure, and we grow dependent on an externally reflected sense of ourselves. Rather than becoming more differentiated as we grow, our navigation becomes increasingly dependent on this externally reflected sense of self, which impedes our differentiation, individuation, and maturation. How we know ourselves (and conversely, how we know the world) becomes more image-based.

We can imagine the ground like sea level, and liken who we are to an iceberg floating in the sea. When we see another, only what appears above the surface of the water is known to us, and if we are not aware of our abstracting process, we identify what we see above water as who this person is. Then we relate to this person as if they had a certain shape and size and dimensions that are real for us, and if our image only reflects the tip of the iceberg, we will relate to this person in such a way that makes a space too small for them. In order for this person to keep the connection they will make themselves small to relate to us. Our image will influence how they form themselves.

The old hag is a manifestation or reflection of an image-based way of knowing ourselves. Embracing what is (process-level awareness) dispels the curse, freeing the life that was frozen, or bound in image, and revealing the innate beauty and aliveness.

Practice, in the sense I speak of here, is not about self-improvement, but rather self-renewal, dispelling the curse of an image-bound experiencing, just as learning to partner with gravity transforms aging into a process of self-renewal.

When we forget who we truly are—boundless consciousness—we are reminded by how we feel—the negative sensations (tension, pain, disease, lack of vitality) and negative thoughts and emotions. However, we also forget what these mean and set out to fix them, which then occupies our energy and attention, rather than seeing them as feedback of mistaken identification with image/object-bound perception. We become caught up in how to fix or hide from the world (our "old hag") rather than seeing her manifestation as an inspiration to wake up from our sleepwalking.

We can't control the conditions and we don't need to. We can, however, fine-tune our alignment with the infinite. This is what I mean by practice. Remembering again and again, freedom and renewal are available with each breath. It is challenging because we live in a world that colludes in taking object-bound experiencing for what is real. Yet it is as simple as an embrace, as the kiss bestowed in fairytales.

Our biology is a reflection of this lived sense of meaning. Just as water molecules can be transformed by love and appreciation (see photos below), our whole being and structure (composed of more than seventy percent water) are transformed by this embrace.

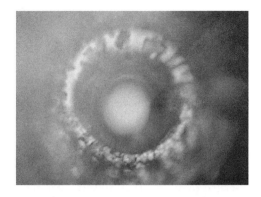

Untreated distilled water

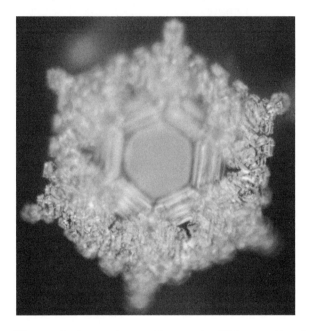

Love and appreciation

These photographs are the work of Masaru Emoto, a creative and visionary Japanese researcher, from his book *The Hidden Messages in Water.*

After seeing water react to different environmental conditions, pollution, and music, Mr. Emoto and colleagues decided to see how thoughts and words affected the formation of untreated, distilled water crystals, using words typed onto paper by a word processor and taped on glass bottles overnight.[8]

Dr. Masaru Emoto's photographs exhibit the effect of consciousness, music, and human vibrational energy on the molecular structure of water, demonstrating how thoughts, feelings, and words shape both the physical appearance of water and its very composition. I see Dr. Emoto's photographs as a beautiful visual display of the unseen: the mysterious and changing structure of water. Though it appears to the naked eye as almost structureless in its fluidity, water is highly structured. And while it has memory, it is very responsive to change. This is beautifully depicted in the photos of the crystalline structure of water before and after it is prayed for, or held with love and appreciation, for example. The photos also show that water responds to music, even when the water is very polluted. Since water covers much of the Earth's surface and our bodies are at least seventy percent water, these visual displays bring home the influence of consciousness, intention, and prayer on both our bodies and planet. I find the photos helpful in imagining potential changes in our structure and the Earth's with the embrace of a loving, nondual attention.

Marty's Story: Transforming Chronic Pain

Marty came to Somatic Learning with a highly-developed sense of compassion for others. As founder and CEO of a very successful company, in his mid-fifties, he struggled with chronic pain, which was sometimes debilitating. During the first year of Marty's practice he effortlessly shed fifty pounds from his large frame, which really revealed just how handsome a man he was. The weight dropped off his body as he learned to receive the support of gravity and stopped becoming concretized in density. A friend commented, seeing Marty run up a flight of stairs fluidly after a year of practice, that he could hardly believe it was the same person he had seen lumbering up the same stairs a year earlier.

Spurs in my neck were the presenting problem, causing extreme pain and immobility, and posing the threat of surgery. This was how I came to study Somatic Learning. I had already attempted all the mainstream as well as many alternative medical strategies. My orthopedic surgeon put me on drugs and wanted to perform neck surgery.

For years my chiropractor worked on my neck. The results were a tenuous balance of trying to keep me out of pain. He helped fix me on a regular basis when the pain got intense. But there was no significant long-term improvement, and I continued to have a need for frequent visits. My neurosurgeon said I might get as much relief through exercise and yoga as through surgery, and suggested I explore that route first.

Somatic Learning introduced me to a new way of listening to my body. I started experiencing myself in a brand-new way. I felt a connection between my silent level of experience and my relational/environmental experience that I'd never felt before.

I can now reflect on all the benefits that took place over many years. First, there was freedom from pain. When pain did arise, the personal relationship to my body that I learned helped me to greet the pain with interest, instead of fear. And when fear was present, it helped me to greet the fear as well. Dr. Kaparo modeled showing up for me on my own behalf again and again when I was unable to show up for myself.

Previously, the differentiation of my feelings was limited to just good or bad, and my single strategy was avoidance of discomfort. What happened was that the line between physical and emotional began to blur, and they all became experiences where I learned to bring in interest and loving compassion for myself.

The Somatic Learning Yoga and Somatic Meditations transformed my chronic pain. The key was how I was participating with myself. There was no line between the somatic work and the yoga. The lessons took the form of the quality of awareness, the letting go, and my ability to allow the wave to carry me. I was sensing myself as movement, rather than as fixed.

Dr. Kaparo's practice affected everything: my relationships, my life choices, and so on. Those were representative of the core change, which was my relationship to myself.

Through this work, I have moved from childhood survival techniques and habit patterns—where I looked to others to reflect back to me that I was OK—to a deeper listening. I love whatever shows up—the depths and the richness in every aspect of my life as I learn to land into myself "like a bird lands into its shadow." There is an undeniable connection and fluidity that has grown in me, between mind, body, and spirit.

Giving value to my silent level of experience has changed everything. Dr. Kaparo continues to model the necessary qualities of love and wholeness, and how we as individuals participate in the process of self-renewal.

Somatic Learning has offered me a portal into myself. I experience my movement from the inside, as if my bones had ears. I experience my relationships, work, play, and time alone from the inside, as a whole new world of listening.

There is a slowing down of my internal experience, a calm, a way that I feel my heart, my belly, my bones and tissues that feels very different. I am noticing when I do violence to myself, and how that feels. I am noticing more when I give myself what I am wanting and feel nurtured.

I am experiencing a comfort inside myself that is dramatically shifting how I relate to people: as if I had been watching a black and white TV all these years, and suddenly I can receive the color signal that has been broadcast all along. I had been looking solely with my eyes, and it is only with all of me that I can see the colors that are actually there. This involves not just the physical "all of me," but an all of me that is truly a vessel for something greater.

Give Birth Slowly

A New Moon teaches gradualness
And deliberation and how one gives birth
To oneself slowly. Patience with small details
Makes perfect a large work, like the universe.

What nine months of attention does for an embryo
Forty early mornings will do
For your gradually growing wholeness.
    —*Rumi*[1]

CHAPTER 5

The Invitation: Birth Yourself Slowly

Let's begin by exploring how we relate to the idea of "practice" to offer the possibility of entering into this practice unlike anything you have done before.

Your practice is the time you create for yourself to give birth slowly. It is an embodiment of leisure, the way you detach from the pressurized field of time. As my friend Brother David Steindl-Rast defines it: "Leisure is the expression of detachment with regard to time." He goes on to say that "leisure … is not the privilege of those who can afford to take time; it is the virtue of those who give to everything they do the time it deserves to take."[2] This is one of the best descriptions of practice I've heard.

The virtue of a daily practice is that we can give everything the care it deserves, and the time it needs to grow into fruition.... Otherwise we find ourselves trying to jump space or we use force to thrust ourselves across the threshold to the other side. However, this force merely perpetuates the tension and violence inherent in the way we are living now ... that keeps us locked into the prison of our experience ... as a separate "self" and as an "object body."

The Practice as Chrysalis

You can use the Somatic Learning practices in this book to hold the field, like a chrysalis, for you to unravel from one state into another ... letting go of "form," of the dualistic orientation of observer and observed, to enter into a nondual realm of presencing. Having a structure, a protected space to contain the experience, is of critical importance. Otherwise you may not feel safe enough to enfold into a more fluid state.

If you were to cut a chrysalis open midpoint, you would not see a caterpillar shedding skin or sprouting wings. You would see a fluid-like substance. The caterpillar actually dissolves out of one state to transform into another. Without the containment, the fluid would leak out and no transformation would take place. Like the chrysalis supports a caterpillar's metamorphosis from one state of being into another, and a womb allows an embryo to grow into a fetus in the amniotic landscape, your Somatic Learning practice can womb you, so that you can give birth to yourself as the embodiment of the vast, unlimited consciousness that is your birthright.

I want to speak to you, dear reader, about how you receive this practice. Employing your will in an effort to achieve some predetermined goal or image turns your determination against you, perpetuating further violence. Our belief that we need to fix or improve ourselves reflects our identification with a very limited image of who we are. If we see ourselves as source, then we would not feel the need to fix or improve ourselves.

We would simply want to live the fullest expression of who we really are, unmediated by limiting beliefs and images.

Dear reader, do not use this practice to perpetrate more violence. Let it end here.

If you receive this practice as a gift, embracing what is with a kind and loving attention, not judging yourself, the practice can be the embrace bestowed in fairytales. It can reveal the inherent beauty of what is and renew you.

Effort

In the very act of reading itself, before you begin the practices outlined in the book, notice whether you are anxious to get somewhere or compelled to read quickly. This is not about acquiring more information or knowledge, but about entering into a deeper listening. *Slow Down.* It is not how quickly you finish this reading and get started; you have already started. The answers are not outside you. Find out what calls to you as you read. In whatever language it speaks … thinking, feeling, anticipation, memory, electrochemically, neuromuscularly, etc.

Please do not struggle to follow my words. It is enough to just to let the words speak to you. You can begin the practice now, listening as a lover to the voice of the beloved.… *Everything I hear … is the beloved speaking to me.*[3]

Simply let gravity draw the meaning further into the silent depths of your experiencing. It is not skillful to tense toward understanding. Nor is it skillful to let your attention go lax, as it will most likely drift into something potentially more interesting … like what's for dinner. Neither does agreeing or disagreeing help. Whatever the state of your body or level of skill or learning when you begin, if you embrace what is actually present without the ambition to change, without tensing toward accomplishment, then you begin in beauty. This was the heart of my beloved mentor Vanda Scaravelli's teaching. Over and over, her basic instruction to me was like a Zen koan: "Learn to NOT do."

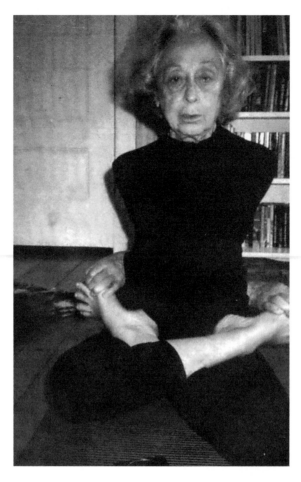

The late Vanda Scaravelli, yoga practitioner, teacher, and author of *Awakening the Spine*

Discipline as a Way of Loving

The embrace is a deeper listening cleansed of all the noise and tensing toward the future, toward somewhere else. We can arrive home, landing into ourselves the way a bird lands into its shadow, filling the space completely. As long as we do not objectify or identify with an image of "self," then this listening becomes a self-sustaining learning orientation. It opens endlessly. Like listening to beautiful music or tasting delicious

Somatic Intelligence Is Your Birthright

food, we do not need to grasp after the experience, but rather to savor it as it unfolds to us.

This is an invitation to enter your practice as Mary Oliver describes in her poem "Wild Geese"—"You only have to let the soft animal of your body love what it loves."[4] As we release our ambition to achieve something, we can practice opening infinitely to love. This is a discipline not in a sense of beating the body into shape, but rather in the spirit of the Sanskrit etymological roots of the word "discipline," coming from the word "disciple," whereby love for the master or the art renders you completely open to learn.

Begin in beauty. This is the practice. It is not that at some point you gain enough skill that your body changes to be more beautiful. As Vanda says, "It must be beautiful in the beginning." These differentiations are offered as a way of slowing down the whole process. In fact, it may feel at first as if the whole world slows down. Then there are many more frames per second of conscious awareness, empowering you to participate in life as it unfolds in the immediacy of this moment.

I have described this process as "self-mastery." While on the outside something may appear solid and impenetrable, from a higher level of differentiation there may be as much space as between the stars, openly inviting movement. However, you cannot get there through doing. In fact, the beauty of the practice is that it makes immediately clear to us how our efforting impedes or constrains rather than enables.

This process of differentiation may become more apparent using an example of auditory intelligence. We cannot sing or play what we do not hear. But if we can hear it, we can with practice grow into becoming the expression of what we hear.

Usually when we try to learn a skill, we focus on the activity or behavior, not on what is taking place inside our own experience. When we shift our attention into our listening, we become aware of the edge of our feeling, sensing, knowing. When we extend our presence beyond that edge, we grow our general capacity to learn, and mastery of the skill comes as a natural consequence.

Finding and Losing Yourself

When I learn a rhythm, playing drums in a drumming circle, the first capacity I develop is keeping the beat. I learn to hold onto the beat in the context of all the parts that the others are playing. But to truly master that rhythm, I need to drop out and come back in, and to be able to find my part in the context of the whole. And so I practice losing my rhythm and finding it again until I can come in anywhere and play my part. This requires much more differentiation than simply maintaining my rhythm once I've begun. So, I do not feel I've mastered a new rhythm until I can find and lose and find myself again and again with ease. This is an essential aspect of the practice.

It is one thing to have a somatic insight that momentarily changes your structure and functioning—which I refer to as a "state-specific effect." It is another to change the course of your life as a whole—which I refer to as a new "general order." As different stresses come up in your life, old conditioned patterns will probably get triggered. You will inevitably lose this new mode of functioning in favor of a more mechanical, habitual mode. When you recognize this, if you don't get caught up in blaming yourself but begin again to extend a deeper listening, embracing what is here and now, a new "beautiful" beginning can unfold. You will find yourself once again poised to ride the next wave with joy and interest. The process of self-mastery will not happen without losing yourself, and finding yourself and losing yourself and finding yourself again. When you remember that losing yourself is part of the practice, you can congratulate yourself for your attention.

> Somatic Learning has taught me what it means to feel both at home in my body and more fully alive in my life. I came to this work feeling awkward about my body and with a restricted ability to express emotion. As I've engaged this work over the last decade I have felt myself to be ever more present in each moment to my physical, emotional, and spiritual experience. This is not to say that I don't lose myself, returning to my awkwardness and

constraint: I do, all the time. Somatic Learning has given me a way to return to myself over and over again, building my faith in my ability to do so ever more quickly. It has and continues to be a truly transformative journey.

—*Margaret*

Developing an Ecology of Affect

The greatest dissipation of the energy needed for transformative learning and change is shame. Really, it's the shame of shame. Each time you recognize that you've lost your connection to what sustains you, or to the flow of joy and interest, shame arises. The affect of shame arises out of our somatic intelligence, before we make it part of our biography (or life story). Shame as affect—the purely biological response—is the way we sense/evaluate/respond to having fallen out of connection with what sustained our interest and joy. It is a gauge that registers disconnect. However, most of us have grown shame-averse in response to trauma and humiliations to our self-esteem. We try to avert the shame by moving away from it—attacking ourselves, attacking another, withdrawing, or avoiding what triggered the response.[5]

When interest follows shame and we drink in our experience, it serves us like good medicine. Rather than paralyzing our learning, it alerts us to having lost the "slipstream" so we can sense our way back into connection with what sustains us. It also deepens our compassion and our connection to all that is, as we sense at the most personal level what any particular condition feels like. This is an important threshold relative to learning. When shame is evoked we will either water the seeds of self-disgust and contempt through our judgment, or we will water the seeds of deeper inquiry and greater freedom and connection. So, if you are looking for places where a shift in your attention will have huge consequences, being awake here will be clearly beneficial, not just for your practice on the mat but throughout the day. Developing a healthy ecology of affect refers to this process of affect self-regulation, not getting stuck in or amplifying the negative affects (especially shame) and returning to or enhancing the positive affects of joy and interest.

There are seven primary affects that are functional in all mammals (not just humans), only two of which are considered positive—joy and interest—in that they support the system in functioning optimally. However, every affect serves a necessary evolutionary function for the survival of the organism/species. In humans, they can co-assemble into complex responses, especially when these affects co-mingle with "biography," or the stories we have become identified with.

Each of the affects can be seen on a continuum from mildness to greater intensity. For instance, when shame is triggered and we become curious about the "disconnect" we feel, we are returned to interest. When we stop "swimming upstream to get away from our experience" we find ourselves floating downstream again—we didn't even have to figure out how to turn ourselves around, because the current naturally carries us. The "relief" we feel in no longer being driven by our shame scripts returns us to the continuum of "joy." As we continue to ride the waves of joy this may at times bloom forth into full-blown enjoyment and even ecstatic experience. Please see the endnote for more detail on the affects listed below.[6]

List of Affects

Positive

1. Interest–Excitement
2. Joy–Enjoyment

Neutral

1. Surprise–Startle

Negative

1. Fear–Terror
2. Distress–Anguish
3. Anger–Rage
4. Dismell

5. Disgust
6. Shame–Humiliation

To summarize, "… an affect is a biological, innate, instinctive response to a stimulus and is fleeting—very brief. It becomes a feeling through awareness and knowledge and an emotion by the additional recall of previous experience from memory."[7]

Donald Nathanson, in his book *Shame and Pride,* succinctly summarizes the impact of these three words: "Affect is biology, feeling is psychology, and emotion is biography."[8]

To support the functioning of our somatic intelligence toward the enhancement of our felt/sense of meaning, it is valuable to differentiate the affective states of experience so we can navigate in the direction of optimal functioning. To this purpose, let's define some terms that will help map the territory with shared language, according to Affect Theory. For developing a healthy ecology of affect, Silvan Tomkins offers this blueprint:

Tomkins' Central Blueprint
   1. Positive affect should be maximized.
   2. Negative affect should be minimized.
   3. Affect inhibition should be minimized.
   4. Power to maximize positive affect, to minimize negative affect, and to minimize affect inhibition should be maximized.[9]

Differentiation

People tend to practice as if the objective is to master a yoga pose or exercise. However, it would better serve us to consider the pose as a learning environment for self-mastery. The mastery of the pose will happen inevitably, as a natural consequence of our heightened differentiation and capacity to extend presence. But the inverse is not necessarily the case. I can hold a pose, day after day, extending the time I hold it, and never grow in self-mastery. As Vanda often reminded me in the early days of my practice, "You're still doing. Do you need to make such effort?" This does not mean giving up and collapsing our attention. The pose can become self-sustaining—without any tensing toward an accomplishment. The koan or apparent paradox of "not doing" and "not giving up" can only resolve itself when we come to a higher level of differentiation in our sensing, which extends our presence.

A great conductor can lead an orchestra because he or she can differentiate the distinctive parts. For instance, he can hear the part of the violins within the context of the music as a whole. His perception of the music has many more dimensions to it than that of an ordinary untrained listener. He can observe particular events within the context of the whole composition. Likewise, in this practice, you will be offered many particulars to differentiate your sensing within the context of sensing the movement as a whole. For instance, in the spinal elongation, you will be encouraged to sense the movements of the diaphragms in relation to the movement of the skeleton in relation to the movement of the soft tissue in relation to the fluid systems, and so on, in relation to space and gravity. As you develop new awareness, Somatic Learning practices will facilitate further differentiation, which will render your presence more dimensionally extended.

Let the yearning do the work. Like a plant yearning for the light, let your yearning to feel the spaciousness open you. As long as it is the yearning that does the work ... without your tensing toward an accomplishment ... then you will do no harm. The longing I refer to is not waiting for or straining toward a "better moment." Paradoxically, this longing is the aliveness that awakens as you begin savoring "what is." In the same way the plant savors the sunlight and grows into the luminosity, your presencing embodies the unbounded spaciousness.

Kabir says this: "… it is the intensity of the longing for the Guest that does all the work."[10]

There is a longing for communion that I believe lies in the heart of all living beings. And it is this yearning that connects us to all that has ever been and to all that will ever be. We get so accustomed to living "without" that we tacitly ignore this longing. Kindle this flame within you and let it have its way with you without efforting.

How to Assess Your Practice

While many yoga, movement, and bodywork practices emphasize alignment, I think it often proves to be a mistake to put too much importance on alignment, because it focuses both on a static image and on the striving toward perfection. And since your structure continues unfolding, the possibilities of alignment continue to change.

Better to rely on the following as indicators of beneficial practice:

- Greater freedom
- Greater aliveness
- Greater flow and interconnectedness
- Greater relaxation and alertness

A Cautionary Note on Pain: Any work that has the power to facilitate transformative learning and change can also prove hazardous if you fail to bring to the practice the proper care and attention.

This is not a reason to avoid practice, because even if you do exacerbate an injury or chronic condition, or expose a latent weakness, as long as you stay with your practice and proceed slowly and carefully, you can transform the unintended consequence of "doing" while practicing the capacity to resolve trauma and heal injuries.

I have often worked with people who have great relief when we practice together, but then they don't practice on their own because they are not sure they are doing it right. However, only in practicing does the necessity arise to fine-tune your sensing, which leads to further learning and differentiation. You have no chance of doing it well if you don't practice.

How do you know if you are practicing incorrectly? Triggering pain or inflammation is the most obvious sign, though like the "idiot" lights on your dashboard, if you are unaware until they signal danger, you stress the system unnecessarily. You want to be listening to self-correct *before* the lights come on indicating that you have strained yourself. This allows for ongoing and gentle self-regulation.

None of the practices should be painful. However, even when you do a new practice well, at times you may feel a different kind of sensation in the soft tissues during or after your practice that lets you know that your system is restructuring. In the beginning, as the muscle fibers lengthen, you may feel a pulling apart of the fascial sheaths surrounding them. Many find this sensation exhilarating—as though you had a great deep-tissue massage. Like an envelope that has gotten stuck together, these sheaths need to pull apart to allow the muscles to lengthen. After a while, these remain in a more fluid state—no longer producing the sensation of shearing or pulling apart that may be present in earlier stages.

How can you trust that your practice is beneficial when you are first learning? Sometimes you may feel sore—as though you have opened spaces that have not been opened or occupied for a very long time. When you recognize the soreness as an awakening, you can savor this sensation—once you are no longer afraid of it. This "soreness" indicates that you have activated a new tonus in your muscles, from having used yourself well or moved something that has not moved in a long time. It is an enlivening, or ripeness, that extends from the bones to the surface. As long as you are not straining you are not likely to hurt yourself. Avoid over-exertion, tearing the muscle fibers through over-stretching the surface tension, or exacerbating inflammation in the joints or tissues that causes pain.

Having said this, I'll add that people are often so frightened by their memory of pain that they back away from their edge. I want to be clear that I am not encouraging you to push through pain—ever—but rather to extend your presence beyond the edge of your certainty or known world. Here, embracing "what is" through a more differentiated sensing may open new possibilities of freedom and movement. You only need to invent/discover a hair's breadth of space through your breathing to extend infinitely.

Fear plays a huge part in perpetuating pain. When we are afraid we tense up to protect against the memory of pain and the intensity of the experience. We will also contract, trying to avoid a future that we have projected the pain into. I have found when I teach the plow, for instance, that people are often frightened by the unusual sensation in the newly elongated tissues of their back as they rest. At some point I discovered a way of alleviating the sensation and began offering the option to my students. I told them that it would be best if they could stay with the sensation and become more fluid, until their form melted into it and the sensation dissolved of its own. What surprised me is that as soon as I was confident in being able to relieve the sensation, they became comfortable opening to their experience and rarely chose to opt out of relaxing through the discomfort themselves.

Some of you come to this practice already in pain, either chronic or acute. Any pain, or what you may come to think of as amplified feedback, offers the opportunity to learn how to self-organize. Learning to move in such a way that does not aggravate pain you might already have allows the organism to heal. Rather than compensating for the constriction, or offering symptomatic relief, this represents fundamental change that enhances the capacity of the organism to renew itself.

Each of the injuries I have personally hosted over the years has helped me fine-tune, by making me more sensitive to how I functioned in relationship to the injured part. For instance, when I injured my subscapularis tendon, it suddenly became vivid to me that how I used my arms relied on my tendons and muscles in a way that subtly strained the shoulder. Through this heightened sensitivity I learned how to do everything I needed to do with my arms—my yoga practice, my touchwork practice with clients, my daily activities—without straining or exacerbating the inflammation in the tendon. Once I learned this, the pain—the amplified feedback—was gone. This is why I suggest that you receive your pain as a gift rather than a curse to be overcome. It is not out of a lack of compassion, nor do I want to romanticize pain. I am suggesting that receiving it as a gift is simply more skillful. The more we can receive it as a gift, the more oriented we are to learn through it the lessons it has to offer, and the sooner we move through it.

This said, it is important to note that if you are using muscle relaxers or pain medication, you need to be even more cautious, as such medication interferes with your ability to sense the feedback through your tissues. This is even truer in the context of your everyday activities. It is easy to ignore the subtler signals of strain and tension before they build up, especially when you are rushing toward your next appointment.

I don't mean to discourage you from doing the practice if you are on medication … just be wise about it. You must start from where you are and not push yourself. But if you don't begin, nothing will happen. You must feel into what is an appropriate challenge for you, and be listening for signs of danger. You do not want to give that responsibility to some external authority, especially one that is not present with you.

Can the damage be beyond healing? I often encounter people who suffer from pain and believe there is nothing they can do that will change their situation because they are too damaged for a subtle shift in awareness to have an effect on them. One way to speak about the subtle shift in awareness we have been describing is to relate to it as meditation or prayer. Both involve entering a receptive mode of being—releasing the tension of "doing" and experiencing gratitude for receiving the grace of the infinite. In this way, anyone can go beyond their perceived limitations from deterministic/dualistic thinking and allow for something far greater to occur. Believe me, miracles do happen!

LISA'S STORY: TRANSFORMING A HEALTH CRISIS

Lisa came to Somatic Learning in her early twenties after suffering the first of several very serious bouts of pelvic inflammatory disease (PID) while living abroad. What opened for Lisa in the process of her self-healing would have been beyond her imagination before, and led her to become a Somatic Learning facilitator herself.

I came home to lick my wounds. My parents knew of Dr. Kaparo's work in Somatic Learning and brought me to her for a session. I was in a weakened state after having been hospitalized and given mega doses of antibiotics. I had had no real experience with any kind of bodywork at that point. After one session, what had felt deadened now felt incredibly vibrant and alive, like the sun's golden rays shining out from my core. My gratitude was immense and my curiosity was tickled. I returned to Europe and to my life there, and it wasn't until about ten years later that I went back to see Dr. Kaparo following several rapid-fire flare-ups of the same PID. The infection had burst out of control and I ended up needing ovarian surgery to save my life, requiring a long, slow recovery. During that time I began practicing Somatic Learning with Dr. Kaparo, learning how to heal and care for myself.

Over time, as I was learning how to be gentle with myself in new ways and to sense into my body's tissues on a subtle level, something amazing occurred. I went to my OB-GYN for a routine follow-up and he felt a lump where my ovary had been. I immediately felt concern: what next? I went in for the recommended ultrasound exam. The technician clearly saw an ovary. "But that ovary was removed last year," I said. "Well, I'm not supposed to diagnose, but that's an ovary. But don't take my word for it. Let the doctor confirm it." The doctor looked down his nose at my chart and declared, without a trace of joy: "You have the very rare ovarian remnant syndrome." But I knew it was evidence of the body's amazing ability to heal itself. I was high on that for months, and still am, really. This is what led me to seek further experience and training in Somatic Learning.

I find that in my life now, Somatic Learning has become like a cherished and constant friend. A fluid practice I could never quite have imagined follows me throughout my days and into my nights. Somatic Learning has become my way of engaging and interacting with the world and myself. This constant friend gently whispers to me, invites me to enjoy space and freedom, whether I am contracted or am bursting with energy. In a given

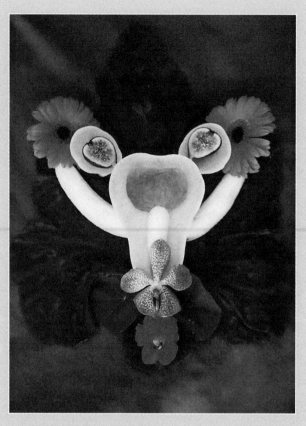

Artwork by Lisa Chipkin, in celebration of her
healing regeneration of her ovary

moment, through one or two breaths, I follow waves, pulses, and flut-
ters of movement as they unfold to reveal precisely where reaction has
manifested into tightness. One or two more, and tightness unwinds and
dissolves. When joy at the beauty and wonder of life overwhelms me, one
or two breaths expand the space in me to receive it, and heighten my
experience of appreciation and pleasure.

Years ago I came to Somatic Learning through the extremity of a crisis
in health. I never knew or expected then that it would become such an
enriching companion on my life's journey.

Research on Wounding and Healing

There has been a large amount of research done on healing in the past twenty-five years. However, because the results are sometimes so varied and ambiguous, and since the criteria for evaluation are not standardized, it may be difficult to draw overarching conclusions.

But I want to introduce you to some of this research now, because I have been very inspired by ideas that have opened up new areas of investigation. These ideas have also helped me to provoke curiosity in people for whom alternative healing methods might have seemed too spiritual or "new age" to engage in, until they saw some kind of data that compelled them to suspend their disbelief, at least temporarily. In some cases, while they can imagine healing working for others, they themselves feel "damaged" beyond repair. It is this kind of insidious underlying belief that I see as one of the biggest obstacles to the flowering of their practice, and so I'd like to share some of the ideas that challenge this assumption.

Embodied mindfulness, or presencing, could also be described by our common-usage word "prayer," by which I mean "drinking in" and "kissing back" the unbounded spaciousness as the beloved. In this light, let's look at some of the research on healing that explores the influence of consciousness on other living organisms, involving the power of intention or presencing that we have thus far been exploring.

One can imagine a long continuum of what is often thought of as prayer. Bowing to all of its many expressions, I am referring in this specific study to the researchers' use of the term "prayer," as it aligns with what we have thus far been exploring: the subtle shift from image/object-level experience to a nondual awareness, as a skillful means to transform pain, stress, trauma, and aging.

It was not until the Spindrift Research Group's studies between 1969 and 1993 that the effectiveness of prayer in different contexts was proven to be statistically significant. Spindrift researchers studied the effects of prayer on seeds, using rigorous double-blind studies, and demonstrated how prayer increased the percentages of seeds that sprouted as well as the amount of their growth.[11]

Since we often pray for people who are unhealthy, the researchers asked, "What if the seeds being prayed for were unhealthy instead of healthy? Would the prayer continue to work?"

To test this question, Spindrift researchers stressed rye seeds by adding salt water to the seed container. The salt diffused upward through the vermiculite, eventually reaching the seeds. The results of prayer were now even more striking: the ratio of shoots from the treated (prayed-for) to control (not-prayed-for) seeds increased sharply, indicating that prayer worked better when the organism was under stress.[12]

This raised the question: "How stressed can the seeds be and still have the prayer be effective?"

The experiment was repeated several times, increasing the amount of stress. "When soybeans were used instead of rye seeds, and when temperature and humidity were used as the stressors instead of salt water, the results were the same: Prayer worked better with increasing stress on the organism."[13]

It stands to reason that if seeds cannot be damaged beyond the powers of prayer, you probably can't be either. In fact, the more stressed or broken you are by life, the more humbled and vulnerable and accessible to the powers of prayer you are likely to be.

Medical writer Larry Dossey, MD, makes the parallel between this and findings from clinical medicine: "We know, for instance, that placebo pain medication—a 'sugar pill,' which has no known biological effect—works better on severe pain than on mild pain."[14]

The Spindrift researchers performed another experiment on soybean seeds to test the relative effects of time spent praying and concluded, "The measurable effect was in proportion to the amount of prayer given, twice as much prayer yielding twice the effect."[15]

The Spindrift studies point to much of what we have learned about the unique potential of somatic intelligence: One of the more remarkable outcomes of the Spindrift research is that there is no loss of effect as the number of parts involved increases. In tests with seeds, for instance, the results were comparable no matter whether the total number of seeds was large or small. Thus, after many years of study, the Spindrift researchers formulated the law of the conceptual whole: so long as the practitioner can hold in his mind an overall concept of the system involved, the effect of prayer is constant over all components.

Whereas focal awareness can only have from one to seven points of observation at a given time, proprioception can bring into awareness an almost unlimited range of sensation. You can have particular points of observation within the context of the movement as a whole. In the breathing practice, for example, you can sense the movement of each of the diaphragms in relation to the movement of their skeletal anchors, in relation to the movement of the soft tissues. How much of the whole movement and how many specific point-events of observation within it that can be discerned are determined by one's level of differentiation. As in the example given previously regarding auditory differentiation, a conductor can distinguish the sounds of all the instruments as they play in concert.

Similarly, beginning students often inquire along the lines of: how do I know if it is happening, or if it's my imagination? I tell them to listen to their silent level of experiencing—to sense what responds to their sensing—since the awareness is not separate from the event observed.

The Spindrift studies also distinguish between visualization and what we have referred to as proprioception. In visualization, thought creates an image that is imposed on or directs the event. For instance, guided imagery such as visualizing a cancerous tumor eaten away by immune cells, or a microscopic broom sweeping the arteries clean, has less of an effect than the power of taking up "what is" in a loving embrace. In releasing the "doing" to receive the infinite, the movement will naturally flower into what it yearns to become. The latter is much more descriptive of what the Spindrift researchers refer to as "nondirected prayer."

Directed prayer occurs when the practitioner has a specific goal, image, or outcome in mind. He is trying to control the system, attempting to steer it in a precise direction. In healing, he may be praying for the cancer to be cured or the pain to go away. In the seed-germination experiments above, he is praying for a more rapid germination rate. Nondirected prayer, in contrast, uses none of these strategies; it involves an open-ended approach in which no specific outcome is held in the imagination. In nondirected prayer the practitioner does not attempt to tell the universe what to do.

Although both methods were shown to work, the nondirected technique appeared quantitatively much more effective, frequently yielding results that were twice as great or more when compared to the directed approach. This may surprise people who favor the techniques of directed imagery and visualization that are quite popular today. Various imagery schools contend that if the cancer, for example, is to be cured, a specific image must be employed as to how the end result will come about. Some studies have suggested that the more robust and aggressive the image is, the better the outcome. But Spindrift's quantitative tests say otherwise. As a result of numerous tests on a variety of biological systems, the Spindrift researchers suggest that healers should strive to be completely free of visualizations, associations, or specific goals. Physical, emotional, and personality characteristics should be excluded by thought and replaced by a "pure and holy qualitative consciousness of whoever or whatever the patient might be."[16]

This inquiry helps to distinguish between differentiated attention and directed attention. I don't think of nondirected attention as the opposite of differentiated attention. What it means to me is that you need to have some felt sense of who or what (as in the case of the seeds) you are praying for. It is not as helpful to pray in the abstract. In fact, the more highly differentiated my sensing (meaning the more acute the listening), the more my participation enhances what happens as it supports the synergy and coherence of energies in our co-presence. I am referring to this work as a practice of prayer or embodied mindfulness, and describing prayer as a matter of presencing spaciousness. Embodying mindfulness, we are a mandala: the union of luminosity and emptiness, as described in Tibetan Buddhism. It is not an undifferentiated attention: it's merely nondual, nondirected, and non-interventionist.

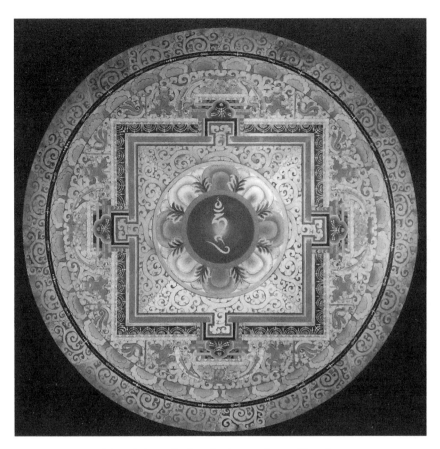

Mandala painting by Lama Pema Tenzin

Engaging Somatic Intelligence in Non-local Healing

The practice of presencing can empower "healing at a distance" through the feedback of your somatic intelligence. Through Somatic Meditations you can learn to engage the feedback—in the here-now of space—in a way that enables you to exercise your capacity to do so in the "not here, not now" aspects of space lacking the immediacy of feedback that our bodies provide.

As discussed in the Spindrift study, such research suggests that it is often our wounding that makes us more open to transformative change. In *The Body Electric* by Robert O. Becker, MD, and Gary Selden, the authors describe many experiments with findings that correlate wounding and the capacity for regeneration. For instance, in humans under twelve years of age, a torn-off finger will invariably fully regrow, if and only if it's torn off beyond the outermost crease of the outermost joint. If only a small part of the finger is lost, it will not regrow, as the signal for regeneration has not been given. This signal is also not given when the wound on the finger is neatly closed by a flap of skin. Several hospitals now follow the regeneration procedure: they sometimes even cut off an extra part and purposely neglect the wound.

Becker and Selden also write about a very interesting link with cancer: As regeneration capability decreases, cancer increases. A cancer on a salamander will eventually kill the salamander: the cancer spreads throughout his body. However, when the limb with the cancer is amputated through the cancer (so half of the cancer remains), the salamander will invariably regenerate: The regeneration electrical impulses make the cancer convert into healthy tissue. Even when this experiment is repeated when the cancer has already spread to other organs, it still works: all the tumors are converted into healthy tissue.[17]

This underscores the importance of awakening somatic intelligence for self-renewal.

In previous chapters I refer to research findings from the sciences of neurology, biology, and psychology that reflect the profound influence of mindfulness on mental, emotional, and physiological functioning. Embodied mindfulness, or presencing, is what I sense the Spindrift researchers refer to as "prayer." In relation to healing, when you practice the Somatic Meditations outlined in this book as an embrace of "what is," rather than in an attempt to manipulate or control something, you will also find the most favorable results. A non-directed or non-coercive approach is what is needed. Simply relaxing is not enough, as you can become too lax in your attention and just "space out." Relaxation is necessary but insufficient. Though better than being perpetually caught up in a stress reaction, it bears only limited results on its own.

The necessary attention involves the two processes of Somatic

Learning: differentiation and presencing. You will find the most favorable response when you are actively presencing—"drinking in" the infinite and "kissing back." The more highly differentiated your somatic intelligence, the more empowered your capacity to creatively and compassionately participate in the unfolding of life. Otherwise you keep focusing from point to point—following, manipulating, or trying to control things from the outside—and never sense the full explosion of life blooming in all directions at once. As in the earlier analogy, you can only sing or play what you can hear; likewise, you can only creatively participate in what you can sense.

All At Once

> All this fires my soul, and, provided I am not disturbed, my subject enlarges itself, becomes methodised and defined, and the whole, though it be long, stands almost complete and finished in my mind, so that I can survey it, like a fine picture or a beautiful statue, at a glance. Nor do I hear in my imagination the parts successively, but I hear them, as it were, all at once (*gleich alles zusammen*). What a delight this is I cannot tell!
>   —*Wolfgang Amadeus Mozart, "A Letter"*[18]

I consider non-directed prayer or embodied mindfulness as that place between "doing" and "not doing" that involves the full engagement of all your faculties. You can't afford to space out, nor should you tense toward accomplishment. Just like Mozart described his process of writing a symphony, you hear it "all at once" and then simply unravel it into form or appearance. Just as he heard all the instruments' voices playing in perfect concert with one another, you must come to sense the inherent resonance and interrelatedness of all your parts playing in harmony. More than that, you must keep extending your presence beyond the known to renew yourself, just as Mozart expressed the dramatic arc of the music within the sounding of every note.

Learning to sustain oneself in "non-doing" requires a sharp attention, as it's easy to fall off the sword's edge of nondual awareness. Paradoxically, this does not require tension but a relaxed alertness. Tension will actually interfere with alertness, and so will laxity. Don't let the energy leak out or dissipate. Keep a tight container around your attention as you practice. Create a specific amount of time and space without interruptions. Breathing deeply, continually stoke the fire of attention to keep it fully ablaze. It is this particular orientation that renders the art and practice of Somatic Learning unique. Its uniqueness is not found in the mechanics of the practices themselves.

Whenever you find yourself waiting—let it be a red flag. There is only now. Learn to distinguish between relaxing and waiting, in which your attention drifts off. Each time you find that your mind has gone astray, don't tug on the leash of attention, because your mind will resist the coercion. Instead, you must become interested in what this moment has to offer you, to take up the gift, here and now, which is the only thing you have.

What I have attempted to do so far is to inspire you to try the practice and make it safe for you to begin. Everything else I have written will prove more valuable when it connects to your direct experience. I invite you to begin now. Begin beautifully. Begin riding the waves of your joy and interest.

Kay's Story: Aging Gracefully

As an internationally recognized author, astrologer, and inspirational speaker, Kay traveled extensively, teaching around the world. Despite being heavily in demand, she always made time to support the needs of her family, friends, and the community at large.

I met Dr. Kaparo on the island of Kaua'i, where I lived for fifteen years. Even though I have enjoyed incredible health and been in good physical shape, from regular walking and dancing, when I began studying Somatic Learning I carried a lot of tension in my neck and shoulders.

I learned that when I began to find my breath and move my breath through my body consciously, new life came in. And it has continued to increase for me daily, while my neck and shoulders reflect this change.

I am practicing Somatic Learning as a prevention and maintenance tool, not because I need to fix some part of me. My focus is on extending myself physically, mentally, and emotionally. I am more limber and free of tightness, stress, or tension than ever before in my life. This wonderful method of honoring the body works in the most amazing and sustainable ways that enliven and renew you, no matter your age or condition.

What I would counsel you to do is practice. Every day, do the practice and the body will respond with aliveness. As my body became more agile and I felt more relaxation physically, my ability to manage and monitor any stress-induced conditions became obvious and immediately correctable.

Now, I love my body and listen to my body and make the necessary changes in my lifestyle that will embrace and sustain maximum physical, mental, and emotional health. Somatic Learning did not change my view of the world. It changed the way I live and move in the world to match the view of life that I believe in.

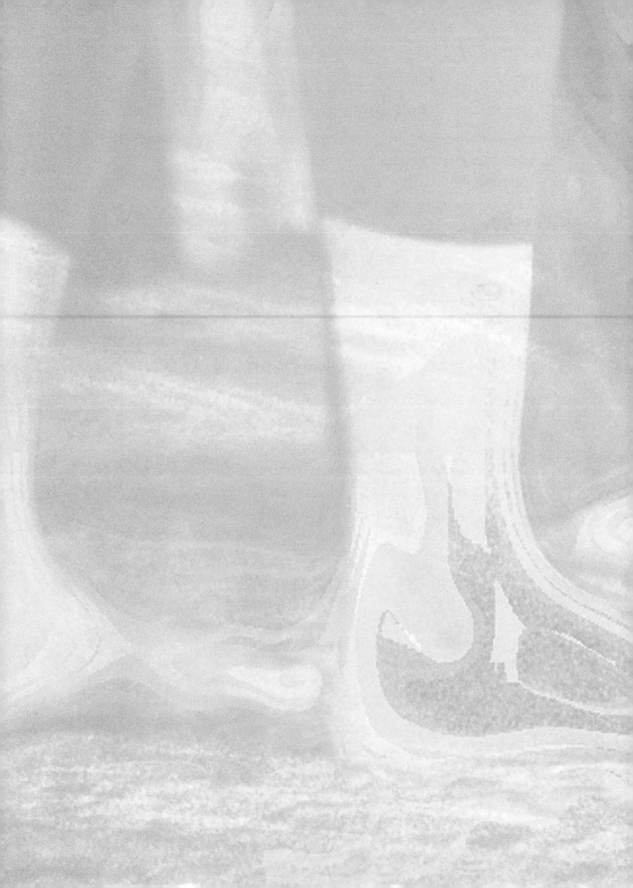

PART II

Reorganizing Your Structure, Reorganizing Your Life

air drawn in after complete deep exhalation little is released in exhale... it is.. released from nose... throughout the body... absorbed...

surfing the wave...

BREATH flows

allow energy to move beyond your structure

sacrum moves down/floats

thoracic inlet

head floats

scapula can fall at same time.

a small amount is released with nose... most distributed

diaphram can be initiation point of pelvis exhalation

Peritenium - like kidneys "empty"

wave goes down legs

SPINE ELONGATES IN BOTH DIRECTIONS

INHALE, feel the suspended spine... energy moves beyond body

Breathing

There is a way of breathing
That's a shame and suffocation
And there's another way of expiring,
A love breath,
That lets you open infinitely.
—*Rumi*[1]

CHAPTER 6

Gravity-Surfing on the Waves of Your Breath

Gravity connects us to all that is. Each breath recapitulates the primordial pulse of life on this planet, connecting us to all that has ever been and will ever be, as time gushes vertically. The French philosopher Gaston Bachelard refers to this as the "autosynchronic moment"—past, present, and future arising all at once. From the Buddhist perspective, when we are present in what I refer to as "the co-implicate" streaming of time, we break the chains of karma. When we open ourselves to receive the unbounded spaciousness with each breath, we receive what truly sustains us. We invent and discover never-ending space, within and without, extending our presence through space like a convergence of rivers. The beauty of breathing in this way is that it "enlightens" our connection to all that is. By drinking in and kissing back the infinite as the beloved, the beloved becomes as intimate as our breath. As one student said after a workshop, we become "liquid love."

> Practicing Somatic Learning for the first time, I recognize the role my skeleton can play in my movements, and I am able to see how fluid I can become. I integrate this insight daily. When I find myself in an 'objective mode,' I can come back into a 'fluid mode.' It is about becoming vulnerable, open, receptive, and giving. Giving and receiving can occur in the same moment: merging and emerging as well. Be present for yourself, yet be supportive for whomever you're touching at the same time. It's really something you have to experience, and I invite you to try it, because it is really so subtle and so beautiful.
>
> —*Tracy*

Like a tree growing our roots into the earth, the deeper we interpenetrate with the earth, the more fluid, strong, and light we become. Gravity draws us to the center of the Earth and as the ground breaks our fall, we receive support from the Earth, rising up through our trunk and out through our crown. As we extend presence, our roots aerate the soil as the amplified wave of energy rising through our spine renews the energy of the heavens. Our arms drink in the energy amplified through the heart center, like branches hydrating the thirsty leaves, and extending through our fingers, expressing this energy outward, kissing back to the world.

We are part of how the universe renews itself ... the undifferentiated wholeness unfolds into form (the explicate order of our embodied consciousness) and simultaneously enfolds itself back into the undifferentiated wholeness (implicate order), ever renewing itself. The theoretical physicist David Bohm referred to this process of self-renewal as the "holomovement."[2]

What is most unique about this practice is the freedom that is possible. Freedom does not need to be an "out of body" experience. In fact, unless it arises in the felt sense of embodied consciousness, freedom will remain limited, like opening a window but leaving the walls intact. One of the unique aspects of practicing Somatic Meditations and Somatic Learning for Yoga is that what we do to enhance our enjoyment of the moment, that presencing or "kissing back," goes beyond simply relaxing our tension and efforting; it actually has the power to transform our physical structure and organismic functioning. The self-organizing power of the practice is like freshly grading the ground. Rainfall can be absorbed equally throughout the soil. It no longer pools or rushes through the old concretized channels, leaving wet and dry spots in the landscape.

Many meditators and yogis experience limited freedom by breaking their identification with the "self" image and the "object body." They may experience pain but not suffer from it; and though they may savor the sense of aliveness or connection to spaciousness, this doesn't generalize to express itself in their movement and structure or organismic functioning. When they get off the mat or meditation cushion, they are often imprisoned in the same dense, restricted, or painful structure, though they may feel less attached to it. They may move through space like a duck out of water, their muscles tensing in an effort to protect against further pain from injuries and trauma. Ironically, even though in the context of their practice they may feel spaciousness and freedom, as they move through the world they return to the same habituations and restrictions that were imprinted in their tissue memory, and with which they are still identified. It is this "image" identification that creates the illusion that our bodies are like objects that we have to propel through space, rather than living portals of consciousness that are continuously self-renewing (by enfolding into form and simultaneously unfolding back into the formless, as illuminated pure spaciousness). This nondual awareness, which we can call somatic intelligence, utilizes the nervous system in a different way, through an open dialogue between its cortical and sub-cortical functioning that expresses itself in each breath.

There is a way of living embodied that enhances our ability to self-sense, self-organize, and self-renew. Breathing is at the heart of this practice … through the processes of presencing and differentiation, we can ride the edge of the wave of our becoming, without getting fixated in form.

Breathing and Birthing

One of the experiences that most graphically demonstrates this embodiment I refer to is birthing. I myself, and many other students of Somatic Learning whom I have had the privilege to support in birthing, have discovered how it is possible to birth ecstatically. Gravity-surfing with each contraction, the mother can elongate her spine, continuously getting out of the way, so the baby rides the waves of the mother's breath downstream through the portal of her womb into the world. Rather than tensing to push the baby out, the mother's intention is on releasing all her tension with the diaphragms at the end of each exhalation, presencing ever more fully with each wave. One mother who had given birth twice before commented as she held her newborn son at her breast that she could hardly believe she had just given birth—the birthing was ecstatic and almost effortless. She felt more relaxed, more open, and alive than she had ever felt herself before.

CARRIE'S STORY: ON BIRTHING

When I discovered Somatic Learning, and how to use my breath within this work, I discovered the universe within myself. In the beginning, I remember feeling fear. My body responded so well to the use of my breath with elongation, I felt like I would change so fast that I wouldn't know how to live in all the internal space I had just discovered.

Becoming pregnant for the third time, I found Somatic Meditations to be an essential ingredient to having comfort and balance within my body.

During birth, I felt so appreciative of all the breathwork and awareness I had developed. My consciousness during labor felt very different than the previous births I had experienced. I could easily breathe throughout labor, and bring awareness to the sounds that formed, both from my mouth and from deep within my body. I still remember feeling how these sounds shaped the inside of me, shaping the birth canal.

Dr. Kaparo encouraged me to elongate with each breath, releasing completely between contractions, and feeling the support as I sensed the wave move through and beyond me.

She supported my perineum while my son came into the world. I remember her describing how my vagina opened and closed during the birthing process with the ease of an eye blinking. Though the physical sensations around birth are intense, I remember the ease with which his entire body, head, and shoulders birthed, in one breath: no tearing.

After birthing my third son, I continued to receive the beauty of this work: the elongations, the awareness, and the gradual rejuvenation I received from the practices. My body today is in a healthier state than it was after I had my first child.

The Pulse of Life

Even in such extreme circumstances as birthing, it is possible to get out of the way, releasing tension and presencing to give birth to ourselves anew, in an expanded state of wholeness.

We start with the breath, the pulse of life, because it is fundamental to everything—all the Somatic Learning practices described in this book, the elongations, yoga asanas, and Somatic Meditations, etc., are extensions of this breathing practice. The practice involves differentiating the movement of diaphragms, organs, skeleton, lymph, muscles, membranes, etc. Let's begin by becoming familiar with some of these structures.

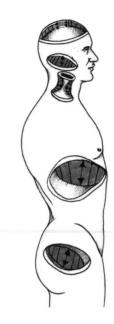

Upper Cranial Diaphragm
Lower Cranial Diaphragm
Vocal Diaphragm
(thoracic inlet)

Thoracic Diaphragm

Pelvic Diaphragm

Locating the Diaphragms

People often think of the respiratory diaphragm (referring to the thoracic diaphragm) singularly. However, we will use the term "diaphragm" to refer to several other muscles, membranes, and fluid structures that define different cavities or areas that move as you breathe, shown in the accompanying figure.

The lowest is called the pelvic floor diaphragm. It extends from your pubic bone in the front of your pelvis to the coccyx in the back, forming the pelvic floor. To help awaken your sensing of the pelvic floor, try performing a few Kegel exercises. (I.e., quickly contract and release the muscles that control the flow of urine and surround the anal sphincter, then relax the muscles completely. This breathing practice does not require a Kegel kind of contraction; I suggest it merely to help awaken your sensing of the pelvic floor.) Once you have located the pelvic floor muscles, slowly initiate your exhalation from here. Just as your abdomen goes in naturally as you exhale, so does the pelvic floor diaphragm, except when you are constricted in the lower part of your torso. When you come to the natural end of the exhalation, (without straining) slowly release the diaphragm and let the breath come to you without effort. The inhalation is not passive, it is very active in the receiving, like savoring a delicious flavor in your mouth. Remember to continually initiate your exhalation from the pelvic floor diaphragm with each breath.

The Myth of "Taking a Deep Breath"

Contrary to popular beliefs about breathing, we don't have muscles to activate an extended inhalation. People say, "Breathe deeply" … as if you could do something to your inhalation that would extend it. This is often misunderstood. No amount of efforting during the inhalation will produce deep breathing. The only way to substantially deepen your breathing is to exhale completely. You do not have muscles of inhalation that allow you to get any more than the top and mid lobes of the lungs filled by sucking the air in more forcefully. The way you can fill the rest of your lungs is by causing them to empty. Like closing bellows, actively emptying the lungs creates a draw from deep inside that causes them to fill all the way to the base—creating what is referred to as a "tidal breath." During the inhalation, the flattening out of the dome-shaped thoracic diaphragm increases the size of the thorax, thus decreasing the pressure in the thoracic cavity. This change in pressure from 760 to 758 mm HG causes air to be drawn into the lungs, like a vacuum.

If you empty the chest first, you will feel like you are out of breath and need to inhale again, even though you have not emptied the full capacity of the lungs. Metaphorically, you can think of it as emptying all the oxygen from the lungs into your bloodstream … so that you can receive the prana (the energy and vitality from the air element) … rather than simply emptying the air from your lungs into the room.

We need only activate the diaphragms, deep intrinsic muscles, and membranes to empty the lungs completely. Then the inhalation becomes effortless. Again, when you come to the end of your exhale (without straining), relax and let the air come to you, effortlessly. In this way you

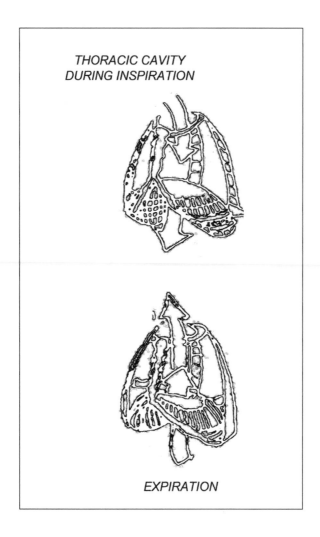

THORACIC CAVITY
DURING INSPIRATION

EXPIRATION

can feel yourself fill, without having to suck breath in. The breath moves through you of its own accord and becomes a relaxed, awakening process.

Activating the Peritoneum to Float the Organs and Skeleton

After we sense the movement of the pelvic floor diaphragm, we want to tune our sensing to the peritoneum. Since the thoracic cavity is longer in the back and shorter in the front, it is critical to activate the peritoneum so that breath is drawn into the back lower lobes of the lungs. The peritoneum is the membrane that lines the back, front, and sides of your abdominal area. It has attachments like leaves, called "mesenteries," that hold your organs so that they can float in a sea of soft tissue rather than being stacked on top of one another. Often we are in such a collapsed state that the weight of the organs atop one another interferes with their movements in relationship to breathing (mobility), with the motility of the organs themselves (the way they move to transport nutrients and wastes, etc.), and with the circulation of the blood around and through them.

Feel what happens as you begin to exhale, first from the pelvic floor, and then along the back—as if you were exhaling from your kidneys. As the pelvic floor moves upward, the peritoneum moves inward. It may feel like a prune, shriveling in the sun. But, instead of making it hard like a prune, let it become more and more subtle until it almost disappears and you become boundless. As these diaphragms move in toward the central core of your structure, sense the way the organs are buoyed by the wave and float upward.

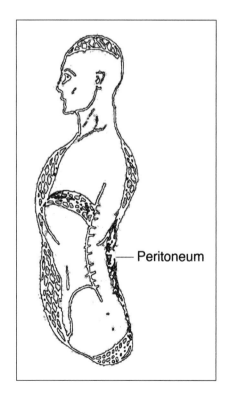

— Peritoneum

As the organs float with the exhalation, the tissues move away from the bones. In this way you "invent/discover" more space between and around the bones. It may only be "a hair's breadth" of space, but that is enough to float your bones. The space opening around the bones is the force of necessity that elongates the soft tissue.

> The brain, nervous system, and heart also give off electromagnetic fields that resonate with our bones and other crystalline-like structures. The crystalline bone structure then amplifies and radiates this energy and information to the rest of the system down to the cellular and subcellular crystalline structures.
>
> —*Gabriel Cousens*[3]

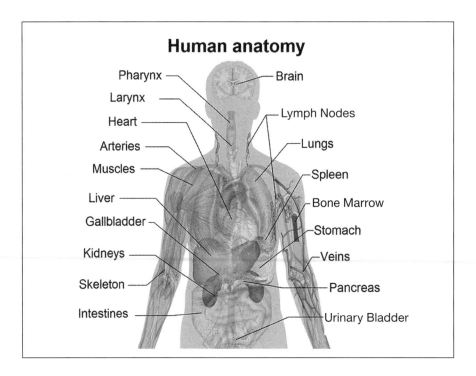

Human anatomy

Pharynx — — Brain

Larynx —

Heart — — Lymph Nodes

Arteries — — Lungs

Muscles — — Spleen

Liver — — Bone Marrow

Gallbladder — — Stomach

Kidneys — — Veins

Skeleton — — Pancreas

Intestines — — Urinary Bladder

Dr. Gabriel Cousens suggests that bones, the only solid crystalline substance in our body, can generate electromagnetic fields and influence our organs, meridians, blood cells, and nerves with these fields. A number of scientific studio studies have shown this electrical-generating ability of the bones, known as the "piezo-electric effect." Taoist practitioner Michael Winn suggested decades ago that "the bones are nothing less than the tuning fork for our whole body. It is the solidity of the bones that makes them such stable transmitters of the deep, rhythmic, pulsating energy that biologically connects our smallest atoms to the primordial rhythms of the stars."[4]

Even while you sit and read this, sense the pelvic floor diaphragm and the peritoneum coming in on your exhalation. And continue sensing up through your back, through the top of the ribcage and into your neck. Also sense from your armpits, from the sides of your throat, through the upper palate of the mouth, the base of the skull, and the top of your head. At the end of your exhale, slowly, gently release all your diaphragms. Savor the feeling of the prana coming to you effortlessly as you relax everything to drink in fully and kiss back—extending your presence beyond your structure.

Sensing the Lymph

It will be valuable to consider the lymphatic system before we begin the actual practice section. The lymphatic system does not have a pump to drive it, like the blood system does. The lymph must rely on the movement of tissues around it to circulate. The lymph is concentrated in areas of greatest interaction between the inside of the organism and the outside, active not only in the functioning of the immune system but also with the absorption of nutrients and elimination of toxins.

For many people as they stand, their rib cage is relatively fixed, and when they move, it moves as a cage. Each rib has relatively little independent movement, thereby constraining the process of breathing. Even in what people generally consider "deep breathing," there occurs limited movement in areas of lymph concentration when the structure becomes constricted in this way. In contrast, when our whole organism is moving in response to the breath, a "sponge-like" squeeze of all the lymph

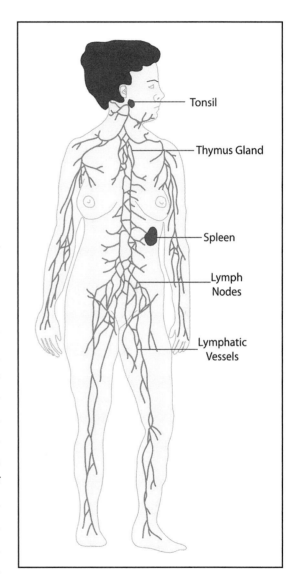

The lymphatic system

nodes occurs, circulating the fluid. Deep breathing thereby prevents congestion and activates the immune system. It delivers nourishment to the cells so they can regenerate and eliminate wastes, preventing toxins from being reabsorbed into the system.

To further understand the movement of breathing, let's get acquainted with more of the diaphragms that are significant in creating intrinsic space. Take a moment to notice the diaphragms displayed in the chart below. To start, we will bring awareness to the three main bowl-shaped diaphragms in the illustration.

Differentiating the Diaphragms

To breathe in a functionally integrated way, every part of our organism must move in relation to the breath. This is rare to witness in "normal" adults. However, look at an infant and you will see the movement of breath not only in their chest and stomach, but in their back and buttocks, legs and arms—even in the soles of the feet, palms of the hand, and top of the head.

As we grow and become habituated, we rely, mistakenly, on our surface skeletal muscles to hold ourselves erect. This interferes with the natural movement of the diaphragms. This mode of functioning is degenerative and self-perpetuating. We feel less support from the ground and have to compensate by tensing our skeletal muscles more.

The diaphragms are areas of maximum leverage for the movement of our organs and skeletal structure. They influence the distribution of our weight and, hence, the force of gravity through the skeleton, without relying on the surface skeletal muscles. The diaphragms also serve as amplifiers that enhance or redistribute the wave function. In a way, you can think of them as amplification modulators.

Three main bowl diaphragms that influence our muscular skeletal structure:

1. the pelvic floor diaphragm
2. the base of the skull
3. the soles of the feet

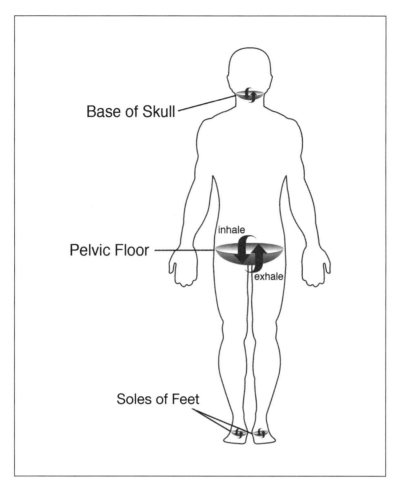

Base of Skull

Pelvic Floor

inhale

exhale

Soles of Feet

The three main bowl-shaped diaphragms that
influence our muscular-skeletal structure

Activating the diaphragms: These diaphragms function interdependently. The pelvic floor, being by far the largest of these bowl-shaped diaphragms, exerts the greatest gravitational pull.... Just as the moon is pulled into its orbit by the gravitational field of the Earth, the smaller diaphragms of the soles of the feet and the base of the skull are drawn into their movement by the larger "gravitational pull" of the pelvic floor. Activating the pelvic diaphragm will activate all the others.

As earlier, initiate your exhale from the pelvic floor and begin to notice how the "moon" diaphragms in the soles of the feet rise subtly as the pelvic diaphragm lifts and flattens. It feels almost like an elevator rising up inside your torso.

Again at the end of the exhalation, slowly, gently release the diaphragms. Notice that the breath can come to you effortlessly and can fill you to your depths without your actively sucking in air.

On the next exhalation, with the movement of your pelvic floor, feel the diaphragms lift at the base of your skull and upper palate. Practice simultaneously sensing all three of these main bowl diaphragms as well as the peritoneum along your back. Practice several breaths until the movements feel smooth and effortless.

Gravity-Surfing and the Practice of Spinal Elongation

The spinal elongation, a foundational practice of Somatic Learning, transforms your relationship to gravity. Instead of having the adversarial relationship of skeletal muscles fighting to hold you up against gravity, you learn how the natural movement of breathing turns gravity into your ally. Receiving gravity's support by reactivating the diaphragms liberates you from habitual muscle tensions that cause pain.

Any use of force, i.e., initiating the movement through a skeletal-muscular effort, constrains the movement of the wave through your structure. What enhances the wave's function is your awareness, the level of differentiation with which you sense the movement and your ability to release habitual patterns of tension that get in the way. You can elongate your spine in any position: sitting, standing, lying supine or prone, in an inversion, and moving through space. If you sit upright in your chair, feet planted on the ground, or sit cross-legged (Indian style), you can comfortably begin these explorations as you read. One key is sitting with your back erect—not leaning against a backrest.

Be aware that the movement of each of these three main bowl diaphragms supports the anchoring of a corresponding bone in an elongation. The anchors amplify the wave so that it doesn't decay or collapse.

1. The pelvic floor diaphragm—corresponds to the sacrum and the elongation of the spine.
2. The base of the skull diaphragm (and upper palate)—corresponds to the occipital and mandibular (jaw) bones and the elongation through the skull.
3. The sole of the foot diaphragms—correspond with the calcaneous (heel) bone and the elongation through the foot and leg, connecting the spine to the ground.

This anchoring is effortless, not muscular. The bones are moved by gravity once the diaphragms open the space. You can think of the anchoring as though someone pulled the base plank off a boat and an anchor sinks down through the water. However, when you extend presence through the anchor, the wave is amplified.

Anchoring the Sacrum

Pay particular attention to the sacrum, named appropriately the "sacred" bone, as it opens a portal to another dimension of movement and presence. Be careful not to tilt or thrust your pelvis forward or back, since this muscular tensing will actually constrain the movement of the wave traveling through your spine.

As the pelvic floor diaphragm lifts, the sacrum anchors the base of the spine toward the feet and the center of the Earth. This happens naturally as the diaphragm gets out of the way. By anchoring, we are not referring to a movement in space, but rather to an alignment of forces.

The sacrum is aligned by gravity, opening a portal or channel through which we can sense our connection to both the center of the Earth and the heavens. As the sacrum anchors, you can sense the equal and opposing force rising up from the center of the Earth as the ground breaks your fall. You can sense this force traveling up through your structure. You can also feel this omnidirectional wave—dividing at your waist. Though it doesn't move measurably through space, the sacrum, by anchoring the movement, amplifies the pattern of waves that extend infinitely in all directions, elongating your spine and opening all your joints.

Gravity-Surfing on the Waves of Your Breath   125

Extending your presence to sense the wave as a whole will enhance the movement, just like a surfer bringing their intention to riding the wave can maximize the ride. You can think of this as *gravity-surfing*—riding the waves of your breath.

Anchoring the Base of the Skull and the Feet

The diaphragm at the base of the skull serves to amplify the wave that the occipital bone (at the base of the skull) anchors—this becomes the ground from which the cranium can extend in all directions like a flower whose petals open to the sunlight.

When the diaphragm of the sole of the foot lifts, the whole foot will root through the ground, sending its taproot through the calcaneous (heel bone). This rooting amplifies the support rising up, as the ground breaks your fall toward the center of the Earth, so you can feel it travel through your spine.

The Exhalation: Floating the Bones

With all three diaphragms active, an omnidirectional wave travels through the entire structure from the waist down through the heels, and from the waist up through the top of the head and arms. Extend your presence to feel the wave flowing beyond your structure, out the arms and top of the head as well as through the soles of the feet, so that the wave is not trapped within the structure, creating a rebounding effect.

At the end of the exhalation, as you slowly release the diaphragms, gradually relax all the tension, receiving the support from the ground as it rises up through your bones. This way you begin each new elongation fresh … holding onto nothing. In this way, surfing the waves of your breath, gravity can deliver you from density and habitual tensions. Presencing is a way to maximize your enjoyment—"kissing back" the infinite.

The Inhalation

This deep relaxation represents the yin phase of the breathing, which we practice more intentionally during inspiration, though you practice this during expiration as well. Feel yourself becoming more fluid as your tension melts into a pool of water. The more you melt, the deeper the pool becomes. I call this "deepening the pool." Then sense the thirsty earth drinking you in, until you no longer exist as separate from the ground. Savor the experience of "drinking in" the air coming to you from everywhere at once.

If you don't feel all that I've described, don't worry. Learn to trust what you DO sense. Stay with what you feel, because from whatever you feel you can extend your presence. The most important thing is not to get ambitious. Muscular effort will constrain rather than enable the movement. The practice is one of differentiating your awareness, not trying to change the body. You must remember one thing: you were born to live in freedom.

Variation: Snake Breathing

In the beginning of any of the practices, especially while the conscious mind is still occupied with following instructions, I encourage you to experiment with snake breathing: sounding on your breath.

Benefits

1. By rendering your exhalation audible, it amplifies the feedback, bringing more awareness to patterns in your breathing ... such as not emptying the lungs completely, holding your breath, using the breath for leverage, etc.
2. Since most people don't do tidal breathing, it's helpful to have a practice that brings the breath back to the spine.
3. Sounding on the breath regulates the speed of expiration of air, slowing it down and making it more even.

Limitations

Think of this breathing variation as a scaffolding to support you in reaching new places in your practice; however, once you arrive there—once you've integrated the new functioning—then you will want to eliminate the scaffolding because it can also limit your breathing. Instead of focusing the regulation of your breath in one place—the mouth (oral sphincter: tongue and upper palate)—you will want to develop the self-regulation of breathing through all the diaphragms working in concert. Eventually you will want to explore not exhaling through the mouth at all, opening the pores of the skin as a membrane even more, and with the tongue resting against the upper palate, opening the throat channel.

Instructions

To your Somatic Learning practice of breathing you will add the element of sound. Exhale as described above through an almost-closed mouth while making the "hissing" sound of a snake at the front of your mouth. You produce this sound by placing your tongue against the hard palate just behind the upper front teeth, barely cracking the lips to allow the breath to escape on sound.

As with the Somatic Learning basic breathing, when you have completely emptied all the air from your lungs, release the diaphragms slowly with awareness, and receive the air flowing into you effortlessly. The more delicious this sensation becomes, the more your presence will extend to kiss back.

Implications

Riding the waves of the breath—gravity-surfing—is the foundation of all the Somatic Learning practices. This practice opens us to more deeply embody the unbounded spaciousness. Each breath is pregnant with the possibility of awakening.

> At the very center of our being is rhythmic movement, a cyclic expansion and contraction that is both in our body and outside it, that is both in our mind and in our body, that is both in our consciousness and not in it.
>
> —*Andrew Weil, MD*[6]

- Awakening to our connection to all life from the beginning of time.... Each breath recapitulates the primordial pulse that sustains life, the same ebb and flow that nourished ancestral life forms, from single-cell organisms to all vertebrates that emerged from the sea.
- Awakening to extend our presence with each breath, opening infinitely, to more fully receive the grace of communion.
- Awakening to the dream dreaming the dreamer into appearance.
- Awakening to the dreamer breathing the dream into appearance.

When I awaken to sense the miracle of infinite love coming to me, yearning for me, I overflow with gratefulness. The fullest expression of gratefulness for receiving the infinite is our fruitfulness, as this union gives birth to new life (the embodiment of boundless consciousness). You are never more than a breath away from giving birth to life anew.

Ron's Story: Moving from Contraction into Pleasure

When Ron, a highly respected chiropractor in his sixties, began studying Somatic Learning, he was looking for greater freedom in his work, music, and life. He was tired of carrying the early trauma he had experienced as a child, and practicing Somatic Learning helped him to refine the tools he was using, both in self-healing and in his clinic, and to become more alive and more fully purposeful. Through this practice he began to embody spaciousness, allowing him to work on deeper levels with his patients. His work evolved into an environment in which he was able to open and free himself while working with others. Instead of compromising his own freedom to support his patients, he began engaging them in a way that more fully supported both his and their aliveness. Here he shares some of the many insights he gained through his practice.

Somatic Learning presents an opportunity to deepen inquiry, freedom, and healing in a supportive environment, with extremely sensitive facilitators.

I find that Somatic Learning clarifies the fundamental issues of perception and differentiation. I have a greater sense of the process of revelation: how insight actually comes to us, not by going over the past and the known, but by opening the space for insight to occur. It may not come of a piece, totally formed, but it comes if we open ourselves to it.

Levels of functioning that were confused by historical trauma congeal in the system and influence how it operates. As we differentiate, the distortions and reactions give way to a new and higher level of functioning, as our body's central operating system integrates. We become more intelligent and more loving as this integration grows.

Ron describes the lubrication that rehydrates the tissues as a very pleasurable sensation.

Pleasure is a wave moving through me that has texture and form. My cells respond joyfully to it. The tissues feel wet when the cell rigidity dissolves.

There is a certain cellular contraction that softens as this transformation occurs. I feel more peace and self-connection, which allows me to more easily include, and truly receive, other people in my life.

I am learning something about seeing that is so crucial, and yet difficult to put into words. I have to keep going back to closing my eyes to soften my attachment to having my mind judging everything. Before, when the two functions of seeing and sensing were glued together, there was much less space inside of me. Now, I feel more expansive. From the outside looking in, it does not seem simple, but it is. It feels rich, and quietly profound. You wouldn't even know how profound it is because it is so quiet, until you actually see how much has changed.

Through this process of differentiation, a freedom occurs. The mind feels healthier, kinder and more alive. It is part of the fluid feeling inside: the cellular awakening. There is a freedom and ease in my structure and in my experience of self. From this place, my old structural inhibiting patterns open up; old trauma and injuries heal, and I am happier and more at peace. Thought is definitely less over-focused: not pushing, more creative. One of the reasons I am drawn to this place is the relaxed playfulness. So much of what I do is serious. I find the playfulness here so attractive. It brings about a feeling of ease and enables me to go into the world with integrity and purpose.

For hundreds of thousands of years I have been dustgrains
floating and flying in the will of the air,
often forgetting ever being
in that state, but in sleep
I migrate back. I spring loose
from the four-branched, time-and-space cross,
this waiting room.

I walk out into a huge pasture.
I nurse the milk of millennia.

Everyone does this in different ways.
Knowing that conscious decisions
and personal memory
are much too small a place to live,
every human being streams at night
into the loving nowhere...
— *Jalaluddin Rumi*[1]

CHAPTER 7

Bedtime Practices

I like to start the day's practice at bedtime—because reclaiming this part
of the day as sacred feels very important. Finding a way to reduce the
residual noise from the day in both one's mind and tissues (experienced as
tension) brings the greatest gain at bedtime.

As we go to sleep, the reduced level of noise will result in a deeper rest. A physician colleague of mine recently showed me the results of some studies: he has been monitoring his patients' as well as his own heart rate variability through a twenty-four-hour cycle. The results showed that the parasympathetic nervous system (PNS)—responsible for growth and repair and immune functions—was most active mainly during brief periods of meditative practice and just after eating. In contrast, the sympathetic nervous system (SNS)—responsible for protection—remained active even during sleep. In healthy functioning, the parasympathetic system should be more active than the SNS, except for brief periods of short-term stress and excitation. Under the stresses of modern lifestyles, we are conditioned to live in exactly the reverse: a sympathetic mode of functioning, primarily being driven into parasympathetic by a full gut demanding digestion. As a result, we are not only stressed most of the day, we continue to "stress out" for the next six to eight hours (a third of our day!) while sleeping, never fully getting the rest and regeneration so desperately needed.

When the SNS is triggered, the blood vessels in our gut squeeze shut, shunting the blood to our heart and large muscles to enable the infamous fight/flight response. This response also channels the blood out of the neocortex (the seat of the conscious mind) and into the limbic or reptilian brain. When our survival is at stake, we cannot afford to be slowed down by conscious thought ... and since the subconscious part of the brain functions so many times faster, we must rely on it.

The SNS serves us in an acute crisis, when our life is actually endangered. However, through misidentification, this stress response has turned into a perpetual mode of functioning. As blood is channeled to our limbs to enable our flight or fight, it shuts down the regenerative, reparative, and vegetative functions (digestion of nutrients and elimination of wastes). This was an evolutionary advantage at one time. When we lived on the open plains and were being attacked by tigers, lions, and bears, it was essential to get out of danger immediately. As biologist Bruce Lipton often jokes, bacteria disturbing our digestion are not as important in that moment as getting away from the tiger. In the end, if the tiger eats us, the bacteria become his burden not ours.

The problem occurs when this response turns into a chronic state of high stress. Back then, when we were chased by a tiger, once we reached safety we relaxed, returning the nervous system to a parasympathetic mode of functioning, which supports, maintains, and regenerates life. Today we are no longer running from tigers. Our primary stress comes from living in shame and fear—resulting from a misidentification with the image/object world, where we react to ordinary situations in a survival mode. One consequence of this state becoming chronic is the general weakening of our immune system, allowing opportunistic, degenerative, and autoimmune diseases to become epidemic. Is your central intelligence (nervous system) functioning like a government that diverts most of its wealth into defense spending, depleting resources from education, healthcare, arts, and social services that support quality of life?

As Lipton points out, whatever part of the budget a government is contributing to defense is not going to social welfare. Just so, with the allocation of our internal energy and resources.

Reallocating Internal Resources—Realigning Your Energy

As in the Judaic tradition, I like to begin my day in the evening—taking the time to release the day and realign my energy, to create a receptive space, to receive boundless love. I believe that at the depths all humans share that longing for feeling our connection with the beloved in all that is. "Living in the world but not of the world," as Krishnamurti liked to say, necessitates that we do not mistake the realm of images and objects for the ground of reality. A continuous realignment with source has to renew our capacity to be in the world while not becoming identified with it. When we go into sleep remembering what we are—love opening infinitely—we are poised toward a lucidity in dreaming and awakening.

The following practices will support you in releasing the tension and habituations we have entrained to. They awaken somatic intelligence—

to participate creatively and coherently in the present moment of sleep or wakefulness.

Evening/Bedtime Practices: 5–20 minutes

The Bedtime practices can be done on a firm mattress or at other times of the day, placing a non-slip mat on the ground. If you choose to practice on the ground, simply modify the instructions accordingly.

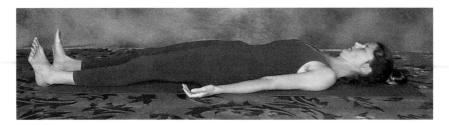

Gravity-Reference Scan

Lie with your back flat on your bed. If this feels uncomfortable, raise your knees. But if you can lie flat for a minute, do so. Take a moment to sense what you notice in this position. Where do you not make contact with the ground? What would the imprint look like if you had ink on you? Notice any differences between your right and left sides.

Now sense your weight distribution. Does your weight fall to the bed in clumps? If you were to drop a sack of potatoes on the bed, certain potatoes would be held up by the others, and some would be held directly by the mattress. Do you feel clumpy? Or to what extent is the weight distributed throughout your system fluidly? There may be some places where it is fluidly flowing and others where it is simply sitting there on the bed. Sense where you are held by the tightness of your musculature.

Take a moment to notice your breathing, just to sense what moves when you breathe without trying to do anything. Maybe you feel it in your belly, or your chest. You might try to sense where the movement ends. Which ribs move and which do not? Do you feel it in the lower back, or the arms or neck, or is it contained within the chest and belly? Sense what moves.

Then notice how you are attending to your experience. Are you scanning it from the outside with your mind's eye—using your visual-perceptual mode? Or can you sense this proprioceptively—meaning through the tissues themselves? And can you sense through the whole structure without focusing on any part, while paying particular attention to specific movements or parts of your structure within the context of the whole? This will reveal whether you have employed your visual perception where it does not serve you best. Using visual perception, you have to track—as though you were moving a scope around you. If you are using your proprioceptive mode of intelligence, you can sense everywhere at once. Because you sense from the tissues themselves, there is no observer, and no object being observed. Notice how you are now sensing this. Do not be concerned if you do not sense everything mentioned here, or if it feels different inside you. Listen to what opens now and reveals itself to you. With continual practice your sensing can open beyond imagination.

Note: While practicing the gravity-reference scan, refrain from making any mechanical adjustments to your structure unless you are uncomfortable. It will prove more valuable to discover ways of self-organizing from the inside-out during the practice. You need to close the door to mechanical interventions (self-management) to discover a non-mechanical mode of self-renewal. For instance: Do not adjust yourself when you notice any bilateral asymmetries. Simply notice them as references to gauge change against later.

Quick Spinal Release

Set-up

Lie supine on the floor or a firm mattress. (You can also do this on a carpet or mat. If you are using a yoga mat, position the bottom of your torso two feet from the bottom of the mat, legs on the floor.) Position yourself such that your outstretched arms can comfortably, with a gentle grip over your head, hold onto a post or the legs of a piece of furniture that will not move. If in bed, use your headboard (often, even if your headboard is solid, you can squeeze your fingertips beneath the frame just below the top of your mattress line). If there are corner posts on your bed, you can lie on a diagonal. Lastly, if you have no headboard at all, you can use the upper edge of your mattress to grip with your fingertips with your arms still resting on the mattress. However, if you do not have firm support from your mattress, we do not recommend that you do this in bed.[2]

Do not strain. If it is uncomfortable to rest the arms on the ground (meaning mat or bed) or if they cannot touch the ground, place a pillow under your elbows to provide support. It is important not to leave the arm hanging unsupported or feeling strained.

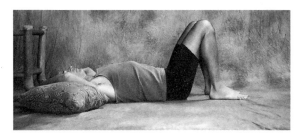

Lying on the floor, using a piece of furniture for the hold

Practicing: The Quick Spinal Release

Lying supine, when you bend your knees so that the feet are standing, the lower back rests on the mattress or floor. This practice supports you in releasing your spine so that even with the legs extended, the lower back rests on the ground.

Instructions

From lying supine bend and lift one knee, as if it were a marionette hanging off a string, placing your foot with your lower leg as close to perpendicular to the ground as comfortable, aligned with your hip. As you slowly pour the weight of your leg through your foot into the ground,

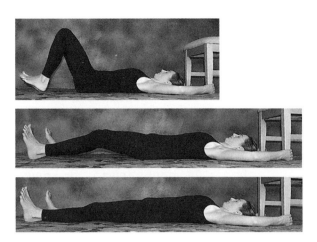

Quick spinal release

especially through the heel, feel the support ripple up through your spine, all the way out your crown.

Resting your lower back into the ground, begin your exhalation from the floor of your pelvis, using snake breathing (making the "hissing sound" like a snake, placing the tip of your tongue on the upper palate while exhaling—especially useful in the beginning of your practice). Often people will hold their breath and use it as leverage to push from, without realizing it. When your exhalation is accompanied by a sound, you will notice when the sound stops. The snake breathing also helps you bring the breath back along the spine. (For more information, see "Snake Breathing" in Chapter 6.)

Do not try to push the surface of your back into the ground, but rather deepen the pool of your lower back by becoming more fluid. Enjoy a few elongations in place, gravity-surfing on the waves of your breath. As the pelvic floor diaphragm lifts, anchor the sacrum, extending the base of the spine toward the feet and the center of the Earth. Invite the wave through and beyond your physical structure. As the diaphragms move, space opens and the sacrum anchors naturally. (Review the instructions for gravity-surfing in Chapter 6 as necessary.)

When you feel ready to move, slowly extend both legs on your exhalation (heels first, flexing the feet, so the toes point toward the ceiling) while gently drawing the support of your headboard or post through your hands and spine. Pour the liquid crystal matrix of your bones down into the ground like salt crystals through an hourglass, especially at your elbows, even as you use the resistance of what you're holding in your hands to draw support though your arms and spine. You are extending your spine on the exhalation, anchoring the sacrum toward the ground and through your feet—as one continuous motion. The legs should not feel like appendages attached at the hip but like fluid extensions of the wave traveling omnidirectionally: down from the waist and up through the rest of the spine, head, and arms. Maintain the connection and flow all the way through, so there is no break. The extension of your spine continues to flow through the extension of your legs.

At the end of the exhalation, as you slowly release the diaphragms, gradually relax all the tension, receiving the support from the ground as it rises up through your bones. Imagine your bones are logs lying in a dry streambed, with rising water causing them to float. Do not begin the next elongation until you relax the entire surface tension, so that you start each new elongation fresh, holding onto nothing. In this way, surfing the waves of your breath, gravity can deliver you from density and habitual tensions.

Repeat the quick spinal release a couple of times until you feel the space open between each of your vertebrae and joints. As your tension melts, sense your fluid presence like a clear lake, and feel the thirsty earth drink you in on each inhalation. As you interpenetrate with the earth, you will come into a much more pervasive extension of presence that is both relaxed and alert. This alertness does not arise from stimulation and can be as easily taken into a deep restful sleep as into a wakeful attention, according to your needs at the moment.

Bring your arms down to your sides one at a time. While keeping your shoulders down, slide one arm along the mat or mattress until it extends out from the spine at a 90-degree angle (we call this "arms on the horizon"). Moving the arm from the horizon the remainder of the way to your side represents a new challenge. Keeping the space under your armpit from collapsing necessitates shape-shifting through your arm. As if you were gliding your hand down through water, use the resistance of "the fullness of empty space" to invite space into the structure of your arm. In this way, the energy releasing from your spine on the exhalation will flow through the open channel of your arm. As the breath flows in, the arms will float gently on the waves of your breath. Then repeat this process to bring your other arm to rest at your side.

Implications

When we use resistance to more fully experience the wave of elongation, it feels like what I see when a butterfly emerges from a chrysalis—the way the butterfly presses against the walls to unfold the wings, drawing blood through them. I have been told that if someone tries to help a butterfly out of the chrysalis, it will never be able to fly and so die. It is in the act of breaking out of the chrysalis that they extend into themselves and emerge fully into their new life.

I have seen the quick spinal release used very effectively during a human birth. I held the hands of one of my students in this position while she gave birth, and she used the flowing support I offered her to extend her elongation, getting even more out of the way ... so that the baby seemed to emerge without strain.

Rest

Pour your bones further into the ground as the soft tissue disorganizes into a more fluid matrix. You may notice as the relaxation deepens with each subsequent breath how quiet the mind is: relaxed, alert, and extensional. As you rest, repeat a gravity-reference scan to notice what has changed since you began.

Getting up from a practice without resting at least enough for the system to settle into a new order—meaning that the structure has self-organized to functionally integrate the new space you've invented and discovered—is a little like preparing the soil, planting the seeds, and leaving before harvest. You lose what you gained too quickly, rather than coming into a new integration.

This is why it is so helpful and efficient to practice a Somatic Meditation before sleep, since you will be naturally resting for the remainder of the night. However, even in the morning you can use the time before rising from bed to extend your presence, to receive the infinite as beloved, drinking in and kissing back—so that when you do rise to start your day, you do so with your energy in alignment with your deepest longing … to live in love, fully awakened in creative, compassionate, and empowered participation with all that is.

Gravity-Reference Scan

Notice what kind of imprint you now make on the ground and any differences from the first time you sensed yourself lying on the bed or floor. Perhaps some parts of you seem more elongated than before or have a different shape. Again, notice the spaces. Is there a different amount of space underneath your neck or your lower back? Underneath your legs? Then notice how your weight distributes itself on the ground—how clumpy it falls, or with what fluidity, as if poured. Maybe this too has changed from the last time you previously sensed.

You might notice what moves as you breathe. Is there any place where the movement is constrained? It may not be externally apparent, but intrinsically, is there any place where your breath seems arrested? Or is it able to flow through your entire structure?

Sense your sensing for a moment. Is something mediating it? Is there an observer and an observed? Or are the movement, the sensing, and the feeling lighting up with awareness without "anybody" watching it?

Variations and Further Differentiations

Placing the Feet for Maximum Elongation

1. When you bring the feet to standing on the mat, open the space between the toes, reaching them out as you place the toes and

ball of the foot down. Now slowly, riding the wave of your exhalation, extend the space between each of the bones along the lateral "spine" of the foot. Resist the urge to put your heel down until you have grown the space between all of the other bones of the foot.

2. This will work much better when practicing on a mat on the floor than on your bed, as the firmness of the ground and the stickiness of the mat will support you in maximizing this elongation of the foot. Notice that when the foot elongates, so does the spine and all the joints, especially in the ankle, knee, and hip. It is best to place one foot at a time. You can use your hand to support the extension and placement of the foot. Since contrast facilitates differentiation, it will prove instructive after extending one foot in this way to place the other foot down normally and sense the difference between the two sides, not just in the foot but all throughout your structure.

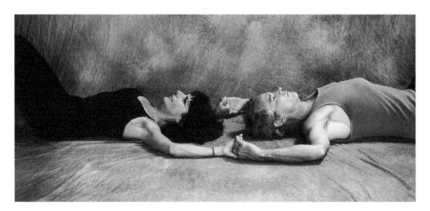

Using a partner for resistance instead of a post or headboard

Instead of using a stationary object to provide resistance for the arms, you can do it with a partner lying opposite you (head to head), clasping your hands together. In this case, using snake breathing will prove particularly useful to synchronize your exhale with your partner, so that you can provide a steady and even resistance for each other through your arms.

Once again: *Do not strain.* If it is uncomfortable to rest the arms on the ground (meaning mat or bed) or if the arms cannot touch the ground, place a pillow under your elbows to provide support. It is important not to leave the arms hanging unsupported or feeling strained.

Variation: Solo without a post for resistance

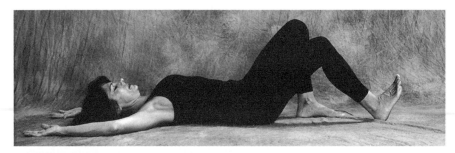

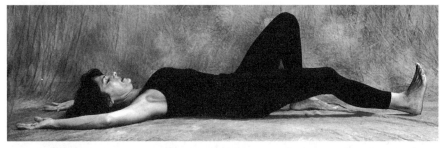

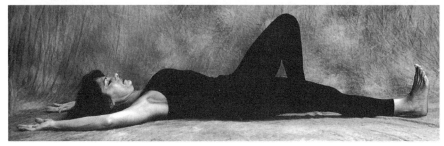

Solo, no resistance, one leg at a time

You can do the same practice without any resistance through the arms if none is available to you. However, in this case, I suggest lowering the legs one at a time.

Further differentiations: *Opening more portals*

If you feel ready to add one more differentiation, it is helpful to sense the movement of the peritoneum.

Once you begin exhaling from your pelvic floor diaphragm, start to empty your breath from your kidneys. You will feel more freedom to release each rib individually—floating them downstream toward your sacrum. This in turn releases any tension that may have constrained the movement of the vertebrae—so that they can elongate more freely. With this additional freedom, you can maximize the elongation of the spine and the support you feel coming from the ground, especially through your lower back. Your lower back will become so fluid that it feels like a pool of water. As you continue to relax any tension you find, the pool will deepen. And as you learn to initiate movement from your diaphragms and bones, the lower back can stay pooled even as you move or extend your legs.

Shape-Shifting Practice with a Ball

Set-up:

You can do this from bed. Or at other times during the day if you prefer, use a yoga mat on the floor. Since it is not necessary to have a non-slip surface for this practice, use anything (as long as it is firm) to insulate you from the cold hardness of the floor.

This practice involves a disorganization of your structure on a tissue level and allows a reorganization that integrates more space through your structure. The shape-shifting necessitates dissolving the identification with the "object body" and a fixed sense of self.

Props

1. Any firm, small ball (not much larger than a tennis ball) or (my personal favorite) a pain eraser ball (with spikes) or a miracle ball that can be purchased from bodywork supply stores.

2. Two pillows for side-lying positions and in case you need one under your head when lying supine.

Cautions

When you first place the ball, you can expect some discomfort, directly from the pressure of the ball against your structure. This pressure may also exacerbate existing tension, bringing it to surface in awareness. It won't serve you to just lie there, "tolerating" the discomfort. In fact, it can even prove detrimental as you begin to further contract to protect from this increased discomfort. Therefore, it is crucial that you engage your full awareness in relaxing as soon as you place the ball. Do not live in a "meanwhile."

You must take responsibility (as with all the practices) for your own safety and well-being. Every time you may have a different proprioceptive response to the pressure of the ball, even in the same location. Only you can know, through your own sensing, what level or quality of sensation can serve as a portal to extend your presence—transforming the experience of pressure into a greater sense of freedom and aliveness. If it doesn't start moving in the direction of "feeling good" as soon as you begin releasing and receiving space, then remove the ball, rest, and find another position that does start to "feel better" as you begin opening and releasing with your breath. Never try to push through the pain under any circumstances. It may be helpful to question your assumptions ... as many of us conditioned in this culture have taken on the belief of "no pain/no gain," which will never serve you in this practice.

Do not place the ball immediately beneath the soft part of the throat, or directly under an acute injury. You can use the ball to relieve discomfort in these areas by placing it elsewhere since the releasing is pervasive, not local.

Drink water before you begin and remember to keep drinking—because as soon as this space opens up, the water will be drawn right into where it's needed most to rehydrate the tissues—you need only provide the water. What a deal!

General Instructions

I am going to offer a suggested sequence of ball placements designed to ease into the practice, as the pressure from the ball will generally increase the intensity of feedback through your structure. As you become more experienced with the practice, feel free to explore where you feel drawn to place the ball, in whatever sequence feels good to you. Or continue the sequence from where I leave off by adding other positions that call to you.

For each position of the ball, place the ball between yourself and the surface on which you lie by rolling off the mat, placing the ball, and rolling gently back onto it. One of the advantages of using a yoga mat is that the ball is less likely to move.

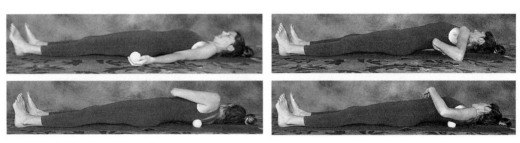

Placing the ball

Begin and End Each Sequence with a Gravity-Reference Scan
Before you switch sides or move on to another sequence, perform a gravity-reference scan, paying particular attention to any differences between the sides. As always, notice any changes from the first and last scan that you did. Please read through all the instructions before beginning the practice. While these instructions provide a valuable reference, you will benefit from listening to a Somatic Learning audio or video to guide your practice. With the support of these resources you may be able to relax deeper into the practice and enjoy being conducted through a gentle, guided facilitation.[3]

Imagine the ball is your beloved. Instead of resisting its touch, see how deeply you can receive it by dissolving from a relatively solid form into liquid, like butter melting in the sunlight. Allow your breathing to change shape—to open around the ball rather than push up against it. Invite the ball to be absorbed into the liquid matrix you are becoming. With each breath, dissolve more of your form and feel the ground drinking up the liquid. Ultimately, both you and the ball will seem to disappear into the fluid matrix of the Earth.

Non-local Sensing

If you feel pressure at the point you make contact with the ball, invite space to open out from there like dropping a stone into a lake. The whole body of water moves to absorb its weight and shape as gravity draws the stone down into the depths. At some point the ripples of movement will settle into a new calmness, once the ball is completely absorbed. It is less about what you do locally—where the ball is in contact with your structure—than allowing it to unravel the order pervasively.

Structures, which ordinarily feel relatively solid or fixed, will reveal themselves to you as movement.

You may start to feel a pulsing, perhaps your cardiac pulse, and as you become more fluid, more subtle pulses may reveal themselves (visceral, cerebrospinal, etc.—you don't need to identify them). As you sense the pulse, it may begin to change shape, elongating, intensifying, coming into a point of stillness, and reorganizing itself. The ground matrix of your tissues may actually change texture and substance ... depolymerizing, etc. As James Oschman's seminal work concludes: "The living matrix or ground substance from which our bodies are primarily comprised is a labile structure capable of displaying all the activities that constitute life."[4]

We don't do these practices to "fix something" but rather to reclaim the present from the old programming, awakening to extend presence on the edge of becoming as the fluid embodiment of boundless consciousness.

SEQUENCES

Sequence One: Upper Torso, Arm, and Head

Lie on your back (supine) with legs bent and your feet standing, or support your knees on a pillow or rolled blanket, so that your lower back rests on the ground.

Position the ball

1. At the middle of the skull
2. At the occipital bone at the base of the skull
3. Between the edge of the right scapula and spine

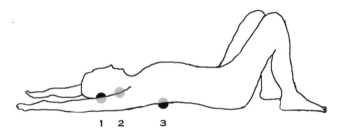

Ball placement, Sequence One

Sequence Two: Pelvis and Leg

Lie supine (on your back) with legs extended. If this meditation follows directly after the quick spinal release, your lower back may feel quite comfortable in this position, relaxed on the ground, even with your legs extended. If you do not feel comfortable you can bend your knees—with your feet standing, or support your knees on a pillow or rolled blanket, so that your lower back rests on the ground.

Position the ball

1. In the middle of your left buttocks muscle
2. In the middle of your left femur bone a few inches above your knee
3. In the middle of your left leg, between the left tibia and fibula bones, a few inches beneath your knee

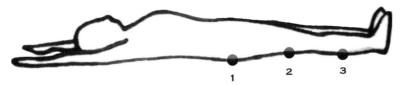

Ball placement, Sequence Two

Sequence Three: Rib Cage, Shoulder, and Hip

Now lie on one side: Place a pillow to keep the head and spine of the neck supported parallel to the ground. Bend the lower arm so the hand rests comfortably at the edge of the pillow, and rest the other arm on your ribs and hip. It is gentler to do the following two sequences on your bed. If you choose to do them on the ground, make sure the surface is sufficiently soft (better to place your mat on a carpet than on a hard floor). Choose the side that most needs attention at the start, then change sides. As you continue the practice on other days, try alternating from which side you begin.

Position the ball

1. At the middle of the hip bone—place a pillow between your two bent knees
2. At the middle of the rib cage
3. At the middle of the thigh with the lower leg extended, bending the other (top) leg—you can place a pillow or ball between the knee and the ground

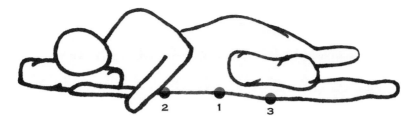

Ball placement, Sequence Three

Sequence Four: Opening the Heart and Pelvis

Lying prone: This position ("lying on one's stomach" or face-down, a.k.a. the prone position) can be problematic for people who have neck injuries. For this and any other reason, if it is uncomfortable just skip it. Generally speaking, lying on your belly will produce the least amount of compression to the neck when you turn your head toward one side, facing your upraised hand with the other arm resting down at your side. Turn your head to whatever side is most comfortable.

Position the ball

1. Between the collar bone, shoulder, and ribs—on the opposite side that you are facing
2. Between the ribs just above the bottom of the sternum
3. Between the pubic and hip bones

Follow your longing as to where you place the ball subsequently....

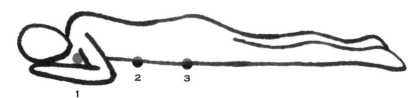

Ball placement, Sequence Four

Implications: Open Dialoguing between the Cortical and Sub-Cortical Parts of the Nervous System

Even though you may begin without any discomfort, it may seem like the side that didn't have the ball begins to "ache with longing" for the openness now experienced on the other side. While you can practice by moving the ball from one side to the other, you may find it interesting to move the ball to different positions alternately, from one side to the other. This allows the "other" side to learn from the side directly receiving the feedback from the ball, while you rest in between positions. Sometimes you may want to keep the ball on one side until the whole area reorganizes around the portal where the ball was placed … for instance, when you have the ball between the tibia and fibula, you may long to place it along the femur, keeping the ball on the same leg until the whole leg releases.

Then as you rest, receive the release directly from the open side on the "frontline" of learning (due to the immediacy of feedback with the ball). Let the "other side" borrow the differentiated awareness from the open side. It is often possible to work both sides at once (as in practicing elongations with a ma roller). However, for this particular practice, I think it will prove more valuable for the process of differentiation to notice the change on one side precisely because it is so different from the other, and then to extend presence by translating the learning to the other side through the process of differentiation, in order to bring greater freedom and aliveness to that side, too.

Intrinsic Connection of the Head and Limbs

Though the "other side" has also become more fluidly connected, it may feel—in contrast to the side the ball was on—as if the limbs are externally connected, e.g., the arm is attached at the shoulder like a doll, rather than intrinsically connected and flowing like a tributary of a river.

Lucidity

We are much more prone to becoming lucid when we go to sleep with the intention of waking up in our dreams to recognize ourselves as the dreamer, instead of identifying with a character in the dream. Likewise, we are much more likely to awaken aware of who we are in the morning—as the embodiment of infinite consciousness—when we go to sleep with that intention.

I have asked many students to pay particular attention to the first few moments upon awakening, and they frequently report that even chronic conditions like pain, tinnitus, depression, and anxiety are often not present immediately upon awakening. This freedom from chronic complaints may only last for several seconds before they experience the community of cells "contract" as they reenter their stories—tightening up and bracing for "the list" (what they have to do that day, their problems and limitations)—in short, re-identifying with the images they hold of themselves and the world. Even this momentary lapse from chronic conditions, however, demonstrates that these conditions are not fixed and unchanging.

The practices help us relax out of identification with how we know ourselves on an image level, because it takes energy to maintain this identification. Like building sand castles at the edge of the sea, we get caught up in feeling the need to protect, defend, and uphold the image/object we identify with, for survival. In this way we react out of fear, activating the sympathetic nervous system.

When we break this identification, we become as free as the ocean itself. Nothing impinges upon us. We are no longer expending most of our energy to protect, defend, and uphold an image of ourselves. Without this chronic drain, we have the energy necessary to stay awake. The flame of consciousness can stay lit.

I strongly encourage bedtime practice, since these are critical moments to extend presence to shift our state of consciousness both falling into sleep and upon awakening in the morning. Since it is possible to be lucid in both the nocturnal dream as well as in the diurnal dream, I invite you to awaken to how you participate in dreaming yourself and the world into appearance.

Note: Before falling off to sleep, read the beginning of the section on morning practice, in order to start off in bed upon awakening.

Morning Practice before You Rise

> The breeze at dawn has secrets to tell you.
> Don't go back to sleep.
> You must ask for what you really want.
> Don't go back to sleep.
> People are going back and forth across the doorsill
> where the two worlds touch.
> The door is round and open.
> Don't go back to sleep.
> —*Jalaluddin Rumi*[5]

Dreamtime Somatic Meditation: A Delicious Transition from Sleeping to Waking Lucidity

Many practices have provided instruction on how to awaken to lucid dreaming in a nocturnal dream. Carlos Castaneda, for instance, suggests looking at your hands and asking yourself if you are dreaming. This Dreamtime Somatic Meditation offers a way to awaken this lucidity in the diurnal dream of waking consciousness. When I recognize that I am the dreamer dreaming the dream into appearance, I can creatively participate in inventing/discovering the reality in which I live.

Of course, when possible, the best way to wake up is on one's own (from organismic self-regulation) rather than from an externally imposed disruption of your sleep process. Even when you must awaken to an alarm, it is best to gently open yourself to meet the day rather than pressurize your reentry.

Just a few minutes here, caring for yourself joyously through this transition, will reflect in who you become as you enter the day. The breeze at dawn has secrets to tell you.

Let yourself dwell as long as possible in your silent-level experience, only gradually activating the discursive mind so as not to lose connection to what is happening at the depths of somatic intelligence. In this way, when you rise up from bed, the surface of your mind is congruent with your silent-level experiencing. The surface and depths are at once reconciled. You have arrived, and you are home. This is in sharp contrast to how most people arise—as James Joyce described one of his characters, "living a short distance from his body."

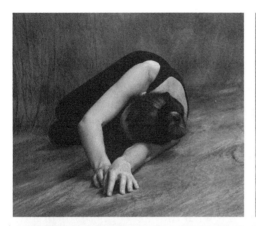
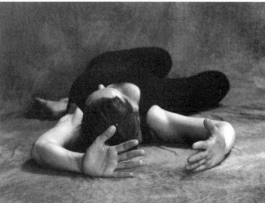
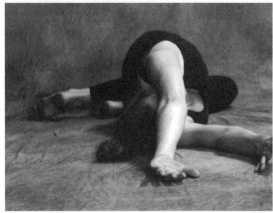

Organic movement in a Dreamtime Somatic Meditation

Instructions

As you awaken, listen for what wants to move and allow the movement to grow organically from the inside out. Don't think of this "stretch" as an exercise. You might want to imagine a cat waking up on the windowsill, luxuriating in the muscular yearnings to reach ... to recoil ... to knead the ground ... to feel the ground pressurize her bones ... ... until she springs to her feet, effortlessly, "hungry to greet the morning."[6] As you extend your presence through the ground, feel the thin lace of your roots aerating the soil and the tendrils of light growing through you, quickening or enlivening your tissues. Lavish the sensation of the "beloved's" luscious touch moving through your breath and being.

Give equal value to the yang phase of the motion, the extension, as to the yin phase, the release and dissolving out of form. Don't look for continuity here. It is like awakening to the pulse of the tides that nourished our primordial ancestors, reflected in our own breathing ... with each inhalation dissolving out of form, and with each exhalation unfolding into form and extending into the beyond. And since the whole can only unfold into itself, you are enfolding back into the undifferentiated wholeness simultaneously as you are unfolding into form, renewing both the explicate order (the realm of form) and the implicate order (the realm of undifferentiated wholeness). This is what the late, eminent, theoretical physicist David Bohm referred to as the "holomovement," by which the whole renews itself.

These instructions may not seem specific enough. My suggestion is that you follow your own muscular yearning. This is an invitation to go to the edge of your certainty and meet the unknown by living into the ambiguity, and finding out how the unknown speaks to you.

Variation

Try the Dreamtime Somatic Meditation from other positions such as free-standing, sitting on the ground or chair, leaning against a wall or partner, etc.

Benefits

The beauty of the Bedtime and Morning practices is that it takes just a few minutes, before sleeping and upon arising, to change the whole quality of your night's sleep, as well as your vitality and presence throughout the day. For many who sleep restlessly or wake up with tension in different parts of their body, these bedtime practices will not only support you in deeper rest, they will also help you awaken relaxed, alert, and renewed. For those who have had lower back problems, these practices may make lying on your back possible once again, though I would not recommend you start sleeping on your back (see note on sleeping positions[7]). Since you are lying relatively still for up to eight hours, sleep represents a point of maximum leverage—where a little attention will produce significant results that improve your well-being.

Some benefits you may experience
- Relaxing out of a sympathetic and returning to a parasympathetic mode of functioning
- Reducing your tonic (resting) level of contraction
- Improving how your weight is distributed and how evenly you are supported
- Increasing the circulation of all your fluid systems
- Increasing your vitality and the mobility and motility of your organs

Before sleeping or arising from bed

As both your nocturnal and diurnal dreaming become increasingly lucid, even a few minutes of reflective writing can deepen "the dialogue with oneself" and anchor your intentions for mindfulness. I suggest you keep a pen and pad for this purpose at your bedside.

Getting Out of Bed

Before getting out of bed, I recommend that you take a moment to repeat the quick spinal release and gravity-reference scan that you did from the evening/bedtime practices.

Once you feel fully awakened, breathing the breath that opens infinitely, your circulation flowing, your whole being flowing in a fluid relationship to the firmness of ground and the openness of space, pour up from your bed in a spiral to sitting. Weightlessly rest your feet on the ground.

Rise to standing by letting gravity draw your weight into the ground, extending your knees while anchoring your sacrum. Have your intention be to release your weight into the earth like a grain silo, rather than thinking of lifting your weight up from the ground. Let gravity do the work for you. This allows the fluid being you are to rise up like upright water. You do not need to re-objectify your body and start moving mechanically. Now as you use the bathroom, and drink a glass of water or hot tea, continue to sense your interrelationship with the ground—rather than moving yourself like an object through space. I would recommend that you wash out your eyes and sinuses, brush your teeth, and change into sweats or other comfortable, loose clothing (preferably natural fiber) for your morning practice.

I do not recommend checking your email or engaging in any of your to-do list before taking at least fifteen minutes for the morning practice. As a parent, I have found it best to wake up early enough to enjoy the solitude of this sacred time. Even in the state of sleep deprivation, the extra twenty minutes I give to myself in this way makes all the difference in the world in my participation throughout the day and with my children. So, in general, twenty minutes of practice will far outweigh the loss of twenty minutes of sleep.

Implications

Wound Healing

The work of Nora and James Oschman on the living matrix has contributed greatly to our understanding of the processes involved in healing and regeneration. They write:

> Microtubules are not the only components of soft tissues that are capable of storing information. A highly respected physiologist has described how records of the ways the body has been used (or misused) are incorporated into the structure of connective tissue. In his well-known book, *The Life of Mammals,* J.Z. Young provides an eloquent account of the

plasticity of connective tissue and its ability to store information.

Young states that the structure of any tissue depends both on how it developed and on the forces exerted on it by other tissues and by the environment. Collagen is deposited along the lines of tension in connective tissues, such as fascia, tendons, bones, ligaments, and cartilage.

Paul Weiss studied tissue cultures and healing wounds, and documented the phenomenon Young described. Wound repair begins with the formation of a clot containing fibrin filaments. At first, the fibers are oriented randomly. As the clot dissolves, fibers that are not under tension are dissolved first, leaving behind a web of oriented fibrin fibers. Fibroblast cells migrate into this web, become oriented along the fibers, and deposit collagen, primarily along tension lines. Any collagen fibers that are not oriented along tension lines are removed by a process similar to the readjustment that took place in the clot. The result is a tissue composed of fibers oriented in the direction that is appropriate to the tensional forces produced by normal movements.

Therapists from many disciplines know that it is beneficial to resume normal use of the body as soon as possible after an injury. Normal motion helps guide appropriate deposition of collagen fibrils. In immobilized tissues, randomly oriented fibers persist and disused muscles begin to stick to each other, particularly where there has been damage or scarring. James Cyriax refers to this as the formation of adhesions, and Ida Rolf calls it "gluing." Both terms describe a random web of connections that form between the myofascial layers of adjacent muscles. This webwork compromises the thin layer of lubricating fluid that normally allows adjacent muscles to slide over each other. When a muscle contracts it therefore tends to drag adjacent muscles along with it, reducing muscular efficiency and precision of motor control.

Disuse or injury promotes a more random deposition of fibers, and this causes adjacent layers to adhere or become glued to each other. Of course, this gluing has a biological purpose: as muscles atrophy from lack of use, they tend to stick to each other, forming a sort of built-in "crutch" to stabilize and support the body.

Earlier in human history when survival was our primary focus, the body's ability to quickly form adhesions enabled us to move sooner to avoid becoming prey. Today we can afford the leisure to allow our tissues to heal slowly and in a manner that encourages complete renewal, eventually restoring our full range of motion. Scar tissue lacks the elasticity of normal healthy tissue, like a knitted sock that has been darned. As a further complication, this irregular tissue then creates a constant source of inflammation. Both the inflammation and the lack of elasticity increase the likelihood of future damage to the area.

Gentle, non-weight-bearing micromovement and touch within the first twenty-four to forty-eight hours after an injury will help prevent the build-up of scar tissue, allowing for new healthy cells to differentiate and replace the damaged tissue.

Soft Tissue Memory

According to James and Nora Oschman, the biophysical properties of the living matrix can explain phenomena that seemed elusive in the past: learning, memory, consciousness, unity of structure and function:

> Connective tissue structure is therefore a record or memory of the forces imposed on the organism. This historical record has two components. The genetic part recapitulates the story of how our ancestors successfully adapted to the gravitational field of the Earth. The acquired component is a record of the choices, habits, and traumas we have experienced during our individual lifetime. The collagen fibers orient in a way that can best support future stresses, assuming that the organism will continue the same patterns of movement or disuse.
>
> It is widely thought that the phenomena Young described are not confined to healing wounds ... Readjustment of collagen deposition takes place in all portions of the living matrix all of the time. This readjustment is the primary method by which body structure adapts to the loads imposed on it and the ways the body is used (see Oschman's article on how the body maintains its shape). Young stated that memories are stored not only in the collagen network, but in the elastin fibers and even

in the various cells found throughout the connective tissue: histocytes, fibroblasts, osteoblasts, plasma cells, mast cells, fat cells, etc.

Young's concept of memory in connective tissues and cells provides a physiological basis for the way the stresses of life, injuries, diseases, muscular holding patterns, emotional attitudes, and repeated unbalanced movements can influence the form of the body. It also explains some of the dramatic effects of various movement therapies. One has the impression that every movement of the body is recorded in the living matrix. Repeated or habitual movements result in a particular connective tissue architecture. Any change in those habits, no matter how slight, will forever alter that architecture.

Intuition and sensitivity have led to practical methods for interacting with fundamental and evolutionarily ancient communication systems in the body. These communication systems integrate and unify structure and function. The integrity of these systems is profoundly important in the healing of injuries of all kinds.

Oschman provides a coherent model for understanding how Somatic Learning and bodywork can open lines of communication, clear the accumulated toxins, restore flexibility, and reduce pain while resolving emotional and physical trauma:

> Biophysics is now progressing rapidly because of a whole-systems perspective. The search for fundamental units is replaced by study of the web of relations between the various parts of the whole. The continuous living matrix, extending throughout the organism, is the context for the web of relations now under investigation. The living matrix has no fundamental unit, no central aspect, no part that is primary or most basic. The integrity of the network depends on the activity of all components, and all components are governed by relations with the whole.[8]

> The world thus appears as a complicated tissue of events, in which connections of different kinds alternate or overlap or combine and thereby determine the texture of the whole.
> —*Werner Heisenberg, 1958*[9]

Joan's Story: Loving Dance Even More without the Pain

I love to dance! I'm often the first one on the dance floor and the last one off. For a number of years I had a knee problem that would not go away. I tried many different kinds of bodywork, years of acupuncture, chiropractic, spiritual healings, supplements, and whatever else came my way: but to no avail. I had to wear a neoprene brace on my knee, and when I did dance I would be crippled for days or weeks afterwards. Then I found Somatic Learning, and after just one session I began to feel some relief. After a series of sessions, I found that my knee problem was completely gone. My posture was dramatically realigned, and my head was once again resting on top of my neck, instead of pushing forward. And yet the practice is amazingly gentle.

The practice develops a trust that the body knows what to do, and invites the body to reorganize itself back to a state of ease, balance, and rightful function. The hands-on work is coupled with home practice, which empowers the client to integrate, maintain, and expand the benefits of the session work. I am ever amazed at the nuances of change that continue, as this work invites more space, ease, movement, and stability into my body. I am forever grateful. See you on the dance floor!

Katrama's Story: Creating Space and Transforming Structure

Katrama was hired as a videographer to shoot a three-day Somatic Learning seminar. She was amazed at how much transformation occurred in her own body as she stood and watched through the camera. After the shoot, she decided to begin practicing Somatic Learning and found the meditations invaluable in reversing structural patterns and habitual strains. How wonderful it was to see her life and practice blossom as her structure decompressed! She had never imagined it possible to create so much change in her structure effortlessly, even when beginning the practice in her late sixties.

I had a profound revelation about my body from practicing Somatic Learning. It is exquisite work, truly transformational. One of my hobbies has been studying dance. I always felt I knew my body and could discern when something was off. Somatic Learning gave me a whole new perspective on experiencing my body. Through the work I became aware of the ability to elongate my body, to create more space and feel the space that wasn't there before.

I never knew until practicing Somatic Learning how spacious I am inside my skeleton and muscular structure, and how my organs float—creating a beautiful choreographed ballet as they work together in harmony. My awareness shifted totally when I developed my proprioceptive abilities.

I felt subtleties of movement I'd never before experienced. The practice enables one to travel and navigate one's body from the inside out—a delicious and exhilarating feeling. I am grateful to have developed my somatic intelligence through this gentle coaching: it realigns my structure, bringing me into optimal functioning.

Today, like every other day, we wake up empty
and frightened. Don't open the door to the study
and begin reading …
Let the beauty we love be what we do.
There are hundreds of ways to kneel and kiss the ground.
—*Jalaluddin Rumi*[1]

CHAPTER 8

Morning Practices

The morning practice is especially beneficial because you have rested and fasted through the night, and the mind is generally more quiet. It is best to begin your practice immediately upon arising, in a time of little distraction from all the intrusions, details, and noise of the day. As Rumi says … "don't open the door to the study and begin reading … Let the beauty we love be what we do."

Set-Up for Morning Practice

When you do your practice, be careful to avoid drafts. If you live in a cool climate that requires heat, my best recommendation is to warm the practice room sufficiently before you begin. Use a non-slip yoga mat, and do not lie directly on a cold surface. These practices work much better on the floor, as the firmness of the ground and the stickiness of the mat will support you in maximizing the elongation and the rooting of the foot. Avoid softer surfaces like your bed for the block elongation as well as the forward bend. However, feel free to practice the child's pose from bed. Socks make the feet more slippery and can constrain the self-organizing movement of the foot, so enjoy bare feet.

You will also need a firm blanket and yoga block (foam, wood, or heavy-duty Tupperware) approximately 4 x 6 x 12 inches. In the event you do not have a block, a blanket can be used instead.

The Morning Practices, 20–40 minutes

Elongation Series

With the term "elongation," I refer to the extensional movement initiated by the differentiated response of the tendons and bones, membranes, muscles, and organs to breathing. The elongation functions at the core of every movement in this Somatic Learning practice.

The elongation series serves as an exercise in differentiation—learning to sense differences. Areas that seem fixed or solid from the outside open as you sense changes and movement from within. Your somatic awareness becomes increasingly subtle as the process of differentiation develops. Starting with a gravity-reference scan offers a point of reference from which to notice change produced by the practice.

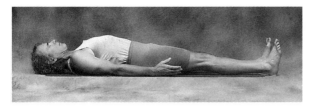

Carrying out a gravity-reference scan from a supine position

Lying supine with legs extended, start with a gravity-reference scan

- Sense how you are lying on the ground. How does your weight fall? What shapes does your body make as you lie there? What size are the spaces between you and the ground?
- Take a moment to sense what moves as you breathe.
- Notice whether you are relying on visual perception to scan your body or if you are also utilizing proprioception to sense from the inside out through your tissues.

Pelvic Position with Block

Bend your knees one at a time so that the feet come to stand on the ground. Sense the wave move through your structure as you raise your knee off the ground. Keep your feet about hip distance apart, placed so that the lower leg is as close to perpendicular with the ground as you feel comfortable with at this time. Now sense the wave of support move through your structure as you lower your foot to the ground. The more fluidly you sense yourself, the more you will feel each movement flow through your whole structure (e.g., even the placement of a foot).

Further differentiation

For maximum extension, elongate the feet one at a time, placing only the toes to ball of the foot down when bringing the foot to stand on the mat. Then while riding the wave of your exhalation, slowly extend the space between the bones of each foot, paying particular attention along the lateral "spine" of the foot. Resist the urge to put your heel down until you have grown the space between all the other bones of the foot. Notice

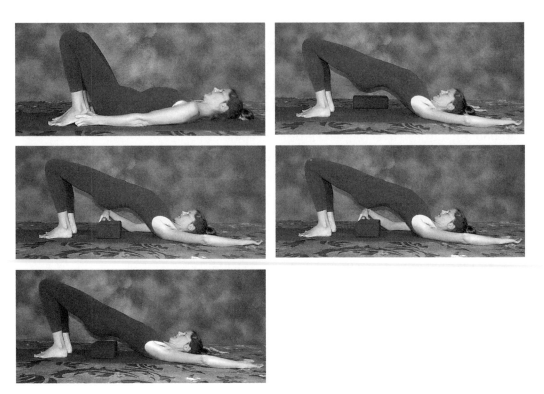

Putting the block into place

that when the foot elongates, so does the spine and all the joints, especially in the ankle, knee, and hip. Before you elongate the second foot, take a moment to feel any differences between sides.

Relax and enjoy a few elongations in this position. Initiate your exhale from the pelvic floor diaphragm while anchoring the sacrum and rooting into the earth through your heels. As the omnidirectional wave goes down, a wave goes up your spine from the waist and flows out the arms and head. When the lungs have emptied, relax all your diaphragms slowly, drinking in the unbounded spaciousness through the breath that comes effortlessly to you. Melt any tension you sense as the breath comes in to begin anew with the next exhalation. As you begin exhaling, kiss back, extending your presence pervasively through space, following the waves of your breath rippling outward infinitely.

Reorganizing Your Structure, Reorganizing Your Life

Placing yourself on the block

When you feel relaxed and elongated, with the next exhalation lift your pelvis and spine up to the base of the neck (at the seventh cervical vertebra) while extending your sacrum to prevent your vertebrae from compressing. Slide in your block, positioning it between your sacrum and the ground, sustaining the lifted position of your pelvis. Start to lower yourself to the ground, one vertebra at a time, from the base of your neck to your sacrum, as you elongate the space between each vertebra on the waves of your exhalation. If you use a blanket instead, keep the blanket in a firm roll without lumps. As you exhale, feel your sacrum and coccyx pressing into the blanket or block. Feel your roots growing deeper, and ground your feet and legs, especially through your heels.

As you feel the pelvic floor diaphragm lift on the exhalation, keep anchoring your sacrum and coccyx. The deeper you extend your presence into the ground, the deeper you will feel your roots grow, like a tree. Can you sense the rooting a foot or two beneath the ground? How deep can you extend your presence?

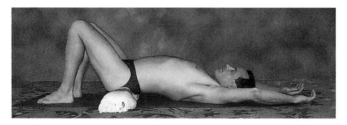

In the event you do not have a block, a blanket can be used instead.

Placing your arms overhead

Before you start the next elongation, bring the arms to rest comfortably supported overhead on the ground. (Review notes in Chapter 7 on how to use pillows if necessary to support the arms.) Take a moment to experiment with differentiating your sensing through only one arm. Pick the one that lies farther off the ground or which has more strain than the other. Pour the liquid crystal matrix of your bones through your elbow as if it were salt pouring through an hourglass. Then sense the crystal matrix of your bones spread out from your elbow through your open palm and fingers as though a night breeze had strewn a mound of sand along the ridge. Do not use your muscles to push your arm down against the ground, as this can accentuate any strain or inflammation already presenting. Differentiate to sense the particular way each layer of your tissue responds to the force of gravity as it rides the waves of your breath. Once you pour the liquid crystal matrix of your bones … feel how the sea of soft tissue reorganizes itself, circulating around the new length of your skeleton. Now take a moment to sense what has changed in the elongated arm and how it differs from the other that was simply lying overhead. Notice if the other arm now feels tighter or denser than the one you differentiated your sensing through. Practice differentiating your sensing through both arms now.

Releasing the ribs

As you anchor the sacrum, practice releasing each of your ribs individually until they float freely, no longer "caged." Imagine them floating out on the waves of your breath like tiny paper boats ceremoniously floating out on the Ganges. Then your lungs can fill without the structure of the rib cage forming a barrier.

Take up every sensation that surfaces, receiving yourself at the depths until the wave subsides. Relax everywhere. Let the breath flow through you, exhaling completely, rooting through the ground. Sense the lymph nodes in your groin, in your armpits, and at the opening of the chest to the neck. Play with flushing out the lymph by squeezing the surface skeletal muscles around the bones in these regions to increase the lymph circulation for cleansing and to support the immune system.

Feel the diaphragms move toward your center on the exhalation. Let the diaphragms take up the weight of your organs, so their weight equally disperses until they feel weightless. It may seem almost as though your insides disappear … and there is only empty space that extends infinitely.

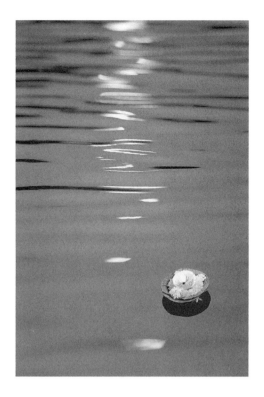

In fact, the boundaries between within and without may also dissolve. See if you can feel this weightlessness from the base of the pelvis all the way up through the back. As you open to the fullness of empty space, feel how your bones extend: through your elbows, fingertips, the back of your neck, and the top of your head. Keep interpenetrating with the ground.

With the next breath, see if you can feel all the diaphragms in the pelvis along the back, and through the thoracic where the chest opens into the neck, both sides of the neck, the top of your mouth, and through the top of the head. See if you can feel all those membranes moving, and at the same time, all your bones. Take one more breath. Can you feel yourself rooting into the ground? Feel how your bones float. The more the membranes move, the more the bones float.

On the next exhalation, gently lift your pelvis up again, rooting through the heels. Keep extending your spine through the sacrum, so that you do not arch your back while lifting. Stay up so that you are resting on your head and neck to seventh cervical vertebra (at the base of the neck) and on the top of your shoulder blades. Pull the block out and return the arms to the position overhead. As you inhale, relax any tension. Learn to rest in this position. Slowly exhaling again, elongate your spine, placing one vertebra at a time on the ground from your neck down to the coccyx.

You can use this opportunity to reorganize your structure as you come down very slowly, extending the base of your spine, through both the sacrum and the coccyx. Continue to pour the cell salts of your bones through your arms and down through the "hourglass" of your shoulders, elbows, wrists, and palms. The arms will polarize the field, providing a soft fluid resistance to support the elongation of the spine. This practice requires an awakened somatic intelligence. Like Lady Ragnell, unless you stop the back-and-forth of attention, your structure will never sustainably reorganize and renew itself—it will simply adjust itself mechanically. You must learn to extend your presence omnidirectionally through both the spine and the arms at once for the restructuring to occur. Any stutter or back-and-forth of attention constrains the opportunity for a new coherence to arise through the structure. In this sense, the reciprocal relationship between the arms (especially the elbows) and the thoracic spine functions similarly to the knees and sacrum (as we referred to in the quick spinal release in Chapter 7).

As the spine elongates, you may feel, in places, as though the curvature turns inside out along the vertical axis. At the same time, extend through the horizontal axis, across your shoulders and pelvis. Use as many breaths as you need, elongating and coming down on your exhalations and relaxing into the place you find yourself on your inhalations.

Do not be concerned if the curves seem to disappear or even reverse as a consequence of the elongation of the spine. This will naturally occur as the spine is extending, and not pose a problem because the spine is decompressing. However, never muscularly effort to flatten the spine on the ground. This can cause compression and may prove dangerous.

When you find yourself completely extended on the ground, bring your arms down to your sides one at a time. While keeping your shoulders down, slide one arm along the mat until it extends out from the spine at a 90-degree angle (we call this "arms on the horizon"). Moving the arm from the horizon the remainder of the way to your side represents a new challenge. Keeping the space under your armpits from collapsing necessitates shape-shifting through your arm. As if you were gliding your hand down through water, use the resistance of "the fullness of empty space" to invite space into the structure of your arm. In this way, the energy releasing from your spine on the exhalation will flow through the open channel of your arm. As the breath flows in, the arms will float gently on the waves of your breath. Then repeat this process to bring your other arm to rest at your side.

Now lower one leg at a time on the exhalation, reaching it out heel first from deep inside your hip. Make certain the sacrum remains extended. Reach the bones of your lower legs out, from the back of the knee and through the heel, as one continuous wave. On the next exhalation extend the second leg, while continuing to extend presence through the first leg. (If you forget to extend through the first leg, you can skew your hips.) On the inhalation, when you feel support rising up from the ground through your tissues, float your bones and gradually relax your muscles. Everywhere that you can find yourself still holding on, continue to release into the support of the ground. Sense the difference between releasing to the support rising through your bones and collapsing. Aside from the physiological difference, sense the difference between this deeply embodied dimensionally extended consciousness and the dissociated state of "dropping out of the body." Don't give yourself away; stay present through your tissues. Practice a follow-up gravity-reference scan (see Chapter 7).

Further Differentiations: Deepening Your Breathing

For women: This practice has helped many women with all kinds of "female" concerns, including PMS, menstrual cramps, fallen or prolapsed uterus, chronic urinary infections, incontinence, endometriosis, fibroids, and infertility, and it can ease pregnancy and birth.

The best place to initiate your breath is from what Taoists refer to as "the ovarian palace." To roughly locate your ovaries, make a triangle with your hands, touching the top of the thumbs and index fingers together. Rest the point where the thumbs meet over your navel and spread the pinkies out. Begin your exhale from deep beneath where your pinkies rest (along the inner side of the back wall of your pelvis) and let the flow of energy move toward your center or medial vertical line, from the ovaries through the uterus and then across the whole floor of the pelvis.

For men: This benefits the prostate gland by increasing the circulation through it. Many men we have seen with enlarged prostates have successfully utilized this simple breathing practice to regain the full functioning and normal size of their prostate gland.

As you breathe, feel the movement of your pelvic floor diaphragm from your tail bone to your pubic bone. As you sense the movement across the pelvic floor at its depth, also sense the wave gently embracing your scrotum and penis as it rises up through your prostate gland on its way to your crown.

For everyone: Imagine that the energy released from the base of the spine with the movement of the pelvic floor diaphragm and the anchoring of the sacrum forms a ball of light that rises up the spine and out the crown of the head. Meanwhile energy pours down through the central channel in the front of the body from the crown through the pineal gland (area of the third eye). With the tongue tipped up to the upper palate, receive the energy that flows down through the throat, heart, solar plexus, and pelvic centers—continue to sense this flow both through the feet as well as rising up through the spine. While you enjoy this flow of energy, deepen your inner smiling, feeling it melt and warm all the tissues through which it opens, bathing you with love and light.

Cultivating Sexual Energy for Self-Renewal

Sense the movement of each breath across your genitals, so that they begin to glow like blowing on embers. This cultivating of sexual energy will increase your sexual pleasure, and can be made available for restorative and regenerative purposes throughout the organism.

Sensing the Omnidirectional Flow of Energy

At the same time that you sense the flow of energy move up from the base of the spine through the crown, you can sense the energy that flows down through the crown, along the center of the body, through the pineal gland, throat, heart, lungs, abdomen, genitals, and out through the root into the earth. You can sense the energy moving down through the earth and up through the heavens, as well as the energy that orbits your own structure … through the chakras, up the spine, and down the central channel. Placing the tip of your tongue against the upper palate while you practice this supports the flow of energy from the pineal gland (third eye) through the thoracic inlet. Some people find it useful to visualize this energy as light, as it reminds them that this movement requires no muscular effort.

Strengthening the Organs

Experiment with initiating the exhalation from different organs. Exhaling from the kidneys to strengthen the chi, especially when you have been experiencing adrenal fatigue, stress, or exhaustion, helps to quickly restore health and vitality.

Notes

1. For yogis: Those of you practicing the upward bow or wheel pose (backbends from supine position) will find the block elongation an excellent way to warm up, rendering the backbend effortless. I recommend fastening a belt just above the knee before you begin the block elongation and then coming up into your first backbend from the block elongation. Rest the head and neck back onto the ground before you remove the block. Then elongate and lower the spine in the same way described above.

2. The block elongation is an inversion. And, unlike most inversions, it can be safely practiced throughout pregnancy and during menstruation.

Sitting Forward Bend (Uttanasana)

Duration: Three to five minutes

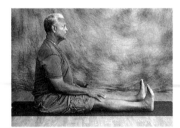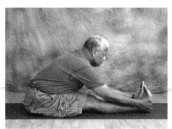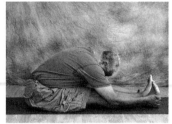

Sitting forward bend

If you can touch your toes without straining your spine or shoulders, then lace your fingers between your toes, starting with your pinky finger between your pinky toe and fourth toe, so that your fingertips can press into the ball of your foot; or wrap your hands around the outside of your foot as shown.

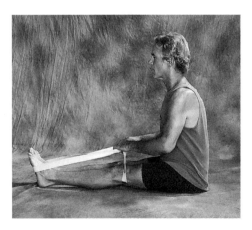

Sitting forward bend using belt

Reorganizing Your Structure, Reorganizing Your Life

If that is not possible at the moment, use a yoga belt (wrapped around the ball of the foot) to give you the extra length needed.

The idea is not to hold yourself up by your hands, which will constrain the movement of your spine, but rather to extend your presence through your arms in a way that completes the energetic circuit, connecting the feet and the arms. The forward bend has two parts. In the first part, we extend the spine to sit more vertically upright, without going forward at all.

Part 1

Initiate the elongation on the exhalation from the bowl diaphragms in the pelvic floor, knees, the soles of the feet, and the base of the skull. As the diaphragms move, you want to glide your bones, as if sliding on the tendons. The surface skeletal muscles will respond, but do not initiate the movement. If you initiate with the muscles, the movement will be bound superficially, and very limited. Feel the omnidirectional wave through your spine, from the sacrum down, rooting through your sit bones and extending the space between the sit bones and the knees, and from the knees through the ankles, and from the heels through the toes. The knee-caps will lift and the feet will flex as a natural consequence of this extension. Be careful not to do this from the surface. From the sacrum up, the wave gets lighter as you de-densify your upper torso and head. Do not strain the arms or shoulders. They should remain relaxed but not limp, extended and connected to the feet, either directly or through the belt. The wave must go all the way through the top of your head and the soles of your feet and hands without losing energy or momentum. When the wave rises through the thoracic spine, the shoulders will fall effortlessly down your back, opening naturally. The wave rising up your spine opens "a hair's breadth" of space between the scapulae (the medial wing tips) and the back. Feel this "updraft of wind" float your wings from the medial through the lateral edges in the fingertips.

Continue to sense the wave beyond the boundaries of your structure, which are arbitrary. This will extend your presence beyond the limitations of the object "body." On the inhalation, relax any residual tension you feel anywhere without, however, letting go or collapsing in on yourself. In other words, do not give up the extension you found during the exhalation, but rather continue to extend your presence, relaxing any tension around your bones. Even your bones will become more liquid, redistributing their mass as the whole breathes in through you. You do nothing. This is an Undoing. You are going to repeat this whole sequence of breaths at least five times slowly, each time beginning from a state of ever-deepening relaxation and freedom.

Part 2

Now, at the end of the exhalation, in the space before the inhalation begins, as the sit bones and sacrum anchor, feel the lift out of your hip joint, like a high dive. Once you feel yourself in "free fall," extend the spine through the top of the head. Do not bend forward from the thoracic spine or head, or lean the head forward.

To open the space in the hips to come forward, two things must happen.

1. You must find more space extending through the knees and the ankles.
2. Your spine must be light. The wave must go through the head to render the spine light.

On the inhalation, you can pour forward from the top of your head, allowing the weight of your head and elbows to stretch the soft tissue passively, without trying to go down. This is important. To activate the lengthening reflex physiologically, you must resist the temptation to stretch the surface skeletal muscles in favor of moving intrinsically, by morphing—disorganizing out of one state and reorganizing into another. Whereas the elongation occurs on the exhale and is initiated from the anchoring of the base of the spine, skull, knees, and heels, the pour forward begins from the top of the head and elbows on the inhalation. Relax any muscular tension you feel, as this pouring forward will round the spine. The next exhalation awakens a serpent at the base of the spine that uncoils, lengthening the spine and straightening the back without lifting the spine up. If you imagine someone laying a board on your rounded spine—at the end of the exhalation, the board would not change angles, but more of your spine would be in contact with it. However, this movement happens intrinsically rather than from the surface. Again, you are going to repeat this breath cycle several times. Each time you can come forward only from the hips on the inhalation, pouring from a straight back into a more rounded spine. This rounding and extending of the spine with each subsequent inhalation and exhalation moves through you like a wave.

Coming up

As you initiate your exhalation from the pelvic floor, use the anchoring of your sacrum as a pulley to draw the spine up. The spine uncoils like a snake, without lifting the upper back muscularly. You must be present in your head and arms so they uncoil with the rest of your spine. If they hang like dead weight they form too much resistance for the wave to support the whole of the upper torso effortlessly.

Sitting Meditation

Duration: Ten or more minutes

This is an excellent time for sitting meditation, now that the mind/body is quiet and alert. You can use your breath as the object of meditation, following the exhalation and the inhalation without trying to control the movement, opening to greater ease and freedom. What your somatic intelligence can bring to the meditation is the capacity to sense the movement of the breath from the inside out rather than to observe from a focal point in the mind's eye. This will allow you to participate fully with your presence, as you do with your beloved, drinking in the sweetness of the divine. And as with your beloved, the embrace is never as delicious as when you are kissing back. See how far you can extend your presence into the infinite following the waves through your spine and the breath. I like to dedicate my practice to the awakening of all beings. You can extend this meditation with the Tibetan Buddhist practice of *Tonglin*. Breathe in to your heart the suffering of all beings, transforming it and sending it out as love and light with your exhalation. When you develop this capacity to transmute such suffering, the suffering that comes up in the context of your daily life feels so small and transient.

When the mind drifts away, bring it back gently, without judgment. Like driving a car, learn how to steer the mind to stay on course, accelerating or giving it more energy when it goes too lax, and de-accelerating or calming it when it gets too excited. It's better to keep the meditation short and bright rather than to extend the time prematurely and practice bad habits when the mind becomes dull. You can start with ten-minute meditations and lengthen the time slowly, following your joy and interest. (For more instructions see "Awareness of Awareness Meditation" in Chapter 11.)

Feeling the Wave
Introduction to the Scorpion Tail

Depending on the time you have available and your level of tiredness, joy, and interest, you can use this meditation to complete your morning practice and come to rest in lying supine, or you can use this as a transition into the LUV sequence that follows.

I have included as part of the Morning practice sensing the wave through the spine more vividly and developing a fluid responsiveness through the entire structure. This way of moving involves a self-organizing of the whole organism as the organs lift and the connective tissue and muscles elongate in response to the movement of the diaphragms and the space that opens between the bones.

This practice can be used to change planes generally between sitting and lying; however, coming up from lying presents challenges that people have the tendency to muscle through as if practicing a traditional sit-up. The tendency arises from the belief that we have to lift our weight against the opposition of gravity and that we need to acquire sufficient strength to

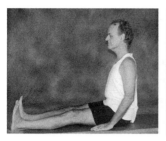
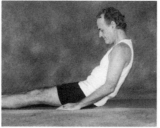
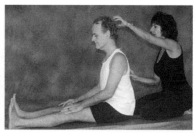

Scorpion Tail Roll: sensing the wave while releasing the spine downward and extending from the base of the spine upward through the head

accomplish this feat. However, mastery of this Somatic Meditation happens from growing your capacity for presencing through differentiation. Therefore, I introduce the first part of this practice here, so that when you come to the full Scorpion Tail movement in Chapter 12, you have developed the necessary differentiation to practice without straining or tensing toward accomplishment.

Downward Roll

Practice this movement on the exhalation. If you roll down and up on the same exhalation it is easier to practice, especially in the beginning.

On your exhalation, release the pelvis slowly so the spine begins to curl down toward the ground from the hips until it is shaped like a crescent moon. Surrendering to gravity, pour yourself toward the ground. Now reverse the wave as you continue to exhale, extending into the ground from the base of your spine and sit bones, and sensing the wave that rises up through the spine as a whole, extending through the top of the head.

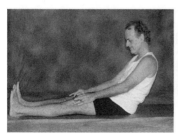
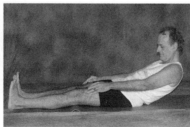
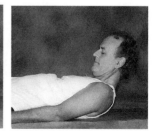

The downward roll is the first part of a larger movement called the scorpion tail (detailed in Chapter 12).

Sense how the curvature of the spine changes as the wave grows through it. Repeat this several times, also noticing how the bones slide through the sleeve of soft tissue of the legs, both as you release down and come up. Each time empty your breath completely, especially from your kidneys, which engages the diaphragm of the peritoneum. Then release the diaphragm slowly and feel the breath effortlessly fill the base of your lungs and up along the spine. Release any residual tension you find in your structure so you can begin anew on the next exhalation. This activates the flow and strengthens the kidney chi or energy. Begin to play with initiating this movement from the flow of chi from your organs rather than trying to control the movement from your surface skeletal muscles.

Gradually deepen the wave, laying more of your spine onto the ground, one vertebra at a time, letting gravity have its way with you. Don't go down more than you can effortlessly rise up when you reverse the wave. Continue to rest completely on your inhale.

Rolling Out to Your Wing Tips and Head

On the next exhalation, deepen the wave downward until the medial wing tips of your scapulae touch the ground. From this point on, you will come into a resting position on the floor, no longer reversing the wave to come up.

Once you touch the ground with your medial wing tips, roll out onto the ground your scapula, shoulders, and arms to the lateral wing tips of your fingers. At the same time, roll out your neck and head. You can roll

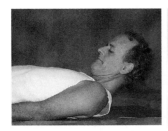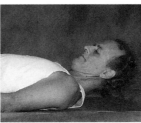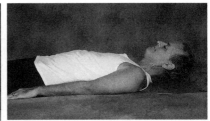

The "wing tips" are the inner edges of the shoulder blades.

out your shoulders, neck, and head just like you can roll out dough with a rolling pin, instead of controlling the weight of your head muscularly.

Rest

Pour your bones further into the ground, sensing the soft tissue disorganizing into a more fluid matrix as you rest. You may notice as the relaxation deepens with each subsequent breath how quiet the mind is, relaxed, alert, and extensional. You can do a gravity-reference scan to notice what has changed since you began resting.

As a reminder, getting up from a practice without resting at least enough for the system to settle into a new order—meaning that the structure has self-organized to functionally integrate the new space you've invented and discovered—is a little like preparing the soil, planting the seeds, and leaving before harvest. You are more likely to lose what you gained, rather than coming into a new integration. Take care in transitioning from this extensional state into your daily activities. Spiral up to sitting. Take a moment to notice how your sitting feels different.

Child's Pose

Since child's pose is one of the most versatile poses, and one that most people can open to easily without struggle, I encourage you to integrate it into your practice immediately. Consider it a resting pose. Since it requires no other warm-ups or special props, you can utilize it as a quick refresher throughout the day when you feel weary or need to release accumulated stress.

Also, because it brings the breath to the spine, this pose serves as a great warm-up before more challenging practices. By awakening the spine to surf gravity on the waves of your breath, you are less likely to strain when you warm up in this way than when you enter these practices cold. Gravity especially assists the anchoring of the sacrum in this position.

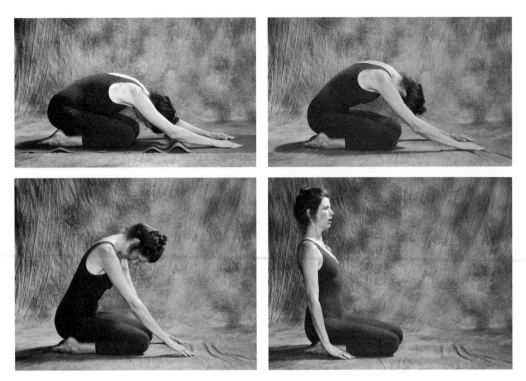

Child's pose and rising up from child's pose

Instructions

Kneel on your mat or carpet, sitting back on your heels, and pour forward from kneeling as you would from standing. Allow the arms to settle into the ground above your head.

Note: If you feel any pain, try adjusting the position using a blanket roll or pillow behind the knee, or between the pelvis and heels, or under the feet, or between the thighs and lower abdomen, according to what relieves any discomfort. If pain resides in the ankles or feet, you can do the child's pose by extending the feet off the edge of a bed (or an armless couch or bodywork table). Make sure you are supported up to your ankles to avoid falling back when you come up. If you can't find a comfortable position, do not strain yourself; work with the other elongations for a few days and try again. You may be surprised how quickly the structure can change.

Sensing the Pelvic Organs

Child's pose is an excellent position to differentiate the movement at the pelvic floor. Take a few breaths to simply feel the movement of your pelvic diaphragm in relation to your pelvic organs, such as the bladder, rectum, and sexual organs. Pay particular attention to the urinary and anal sphincters. Try tensing and then incrementally releasing the tension into complete relaxation. Women: This is an excellent position for practicing Kegels. Sense how the movement changes when you relax these organs one at a time.

As you initiate your exhalation from the pelvic floor diaphragm, sense how it peels away from the anchoring sacrum and coccyx, like one river diverging into two. Sense the way the pelvic organs and tissues float on the flow of these rivers.

Feel the swirling vortexes of this fluid movement around each of your sit bones. These swirls clear any congestion in the pelvis, in the same way the flow of water clears debris from the riverbanks. Sense how these little energy whirlpools open space in your hip joints and de-densify the pelvis.

Dissolve into the wave as it goes beyond your structure and opens infinitely, presencing and kissing back. Allow gravity to liberate you, through

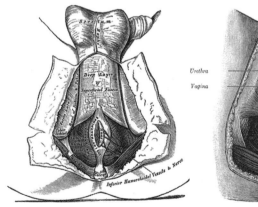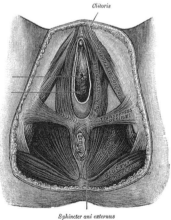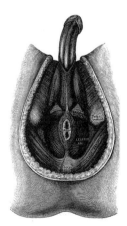

View from pelvic floor, male and female

the wave, rather than trying to extend your structure with force. Sense the bones moving through a sea of soft tissue on the exhalation before the thirsty ground absorbs the ocean you have become on the inhalation.

Use the anchoring of the calcaneous, sacrum, and occiput like a stake in the ground or a magnetic pole to re-polarize the field. Think of yourself as frequency in resonance. Rather than sensing yourself at an object level, play with sensing yourself as very fine bits of matter surrounded by empty space. Let the dynamics of attention reconstitute you—like iron filings drawn toward a magnet.

Follow the "Coming up" instructions from the sitting forward bend (please see page 179) to pour up. Enjoy a few breaths of rest while doing a gravity-reference scan in this position before spiraling down to rest further or up to standing.

Implications

Child's pose can serve very well as a counter pose, especially for inversions like headstand, bacasana, and scorpion, as it releases any pressure or tension from the neck and head. To get into child's pose from an inversion, simply lower your pelvis over your heels as you anchor the sacrum and ride the elongation out through your upper spine and arms. Remember to anchor the wave through the arms, especially at the elbows and wrists, as well as through the base of the skull.

LUV Sequence

If you are beginning your practice here, start with a gravity-reference scan, lying supine; otherwise, just continue.

Forming the L

Take a moment to sense the breath initiating from the ovarian palace or the back of the pelvic bowl (as described in the pelvic position elongation with block, above—the first exercise in this chapter). When you initiate the movement of the pelvic floor diaphragm from here, rather than from

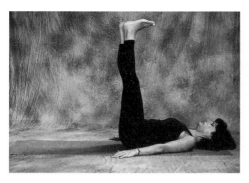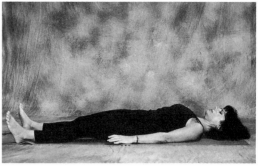

Starting from the gravity-reference scan, the "L" position

the surface of the pelvic floor, you enjoy much greater support from the diaphragm. This will release the sacrum and the feet, to anchor down as the pelvic diaphragm clears the way. It will also allow you to extend the tailbone from the sacrum to maximize the flow of energy from the base of the spine. Take a few breaths until your reproductive organs feel enlivened, as though someone had blown on embers to make them glow. Finding this deep initiation of the breath enables you to tap into a source of power far beyond muscular strength, as if you were tapping into the vertebrate imagination of the whole species … calling forth the power of your ancestors now…. And it will come to you because at this moment you are the only reason your ancestors ever existed.

Bend the knees and bring the feet to standing, deepening the pool of your lower back. On the exhalation, let the feet rise up from the pelvis as if you were sliding them up against a wall, until your legs rest perpendicular to the ground.

Extend the femur out of the hip joint, extend the tibia/fibula out of the knee joint, and extend the spine of the foot so that the legs feel weightless and do not require a lot of tensing to hold them up. Enjoy several breaths. On the inhalation, relax everything, while sustaining the extension through your structure. On each exhalation begin elongating the spine, riding the waves of the breath. You can press your legs into an invisible wall to further the extension of your hips and spine.

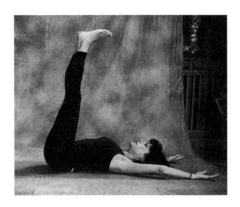

Extended "L" position

Lift your arms, forming an arc to rest on the ground above the head, while pouring the shoulders into the ground. As you sense the vertical axis of the wave traveling through your structure (elongating your spine), sense the wave flowing along your horizontal axis as well, extending through your shoulders and out the arms. Pour the liquid crystalline matrix of your bones into the ground through your shoulders, elbows, and palms as if they were salt crystals pouring through an hourglass.

Forming the "U"

As you continue releasing your lower back and shoulders into the ground, move your arms like spokes of a wheel from the center or shoulder, so that the fingertips extend toward the ceiling with your arms standing

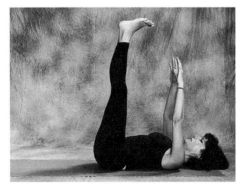

The "U" position

Reorganizing Your Structure, Reorganizing Your Life

perpendicular to the ground and parallel to your legs. Elongate the spine for several breaths in this position so that you feel both the horizontal and vertical waves moving through the spine and the extremities.

Forming the "V"

Bringing the legs together and keeping the knees and elbows extended, gently grasp your toes with your hands. And if you can't reach your toes without straining, you can hold the back of your ankles or legs (anywhere except at the knee—so as not to encourage them to bend). It is critical to not lift the shoulders; rather, keep pouring them into the ground.

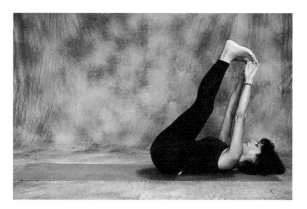

Grasping the feet

The arms and legs provide resistance to each other. The legs supply resistance to support the shoulders rolling back and down into the ground; and the arms provide resistance to anchor the coccyx into the ground.

Open the legs slowly out into a "V," extending the legs up and out of the hip sockets, so that the legs never fall or collapse in the hip joint. Do not try to stretch the surface skeletal muscles.

If you feel like you're holding yourself up from your arms, relax your muscles and elongate your spine, reaching out from all your joints. This will also release any quivering that may occur when your muscles are overstretched. This will activate the lengthening reflex physiologically

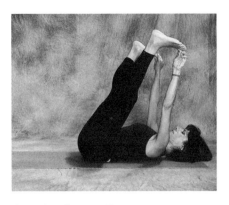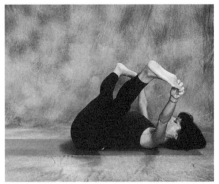

Opening into "V"

rather than the stretching reflex, and your muscle fibers will lengthen rather than pull on the surface.

Bring the legs back together, initiating the breath from the ovarian palace or as described above for men. All of this movement should be on the exhalation. Use the inhalation to relax and extend your presence through the structure and beyond.

Let go of your hands and re-extend the arms and legs into the "U" position. Enjoy a few breaths. Slowly release the arms back down overhead, returning to the "L" position, pouring the liquid matrix of the bones into the ground. Elongate a few times here, then sense what has changed from the first time you were lying in this position.

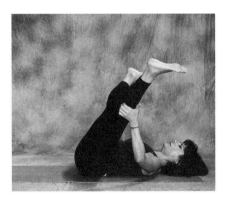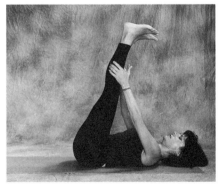

Alternative hold. It is more important to not strain than to grasp the toes.

Lowering the legs

Bring the knees bent into the chest. Then continue to deepen the pool of your lower back as you lower your feet to the ground so that they land ball of the foot first and then extend through the heels. Enjoy a few elongations in this position before extending the legs to the ground, one at a time, as in the pelvic position with block elongation above.

LUV Pose Variations

Enhancing tonus, healing, and immune functions: Soft-bellied shimmy shake

From the "U" position

If the mobility and the motility of the organs are constrained, the tone of the soft tissue will reflect the lack of vitality in the organs. Even if you work out, you can harden these muscles, but you will not revitalize the tonus, the energy imbued from the core, without liberating the breath and the resultant flow of energy from the organs.

In a healthy state of functioning, the organs move freely both to metabolize nourishment and waste as well as in relationship to breathing and our movement in space. Since the energy flows freely through these movements, it imbues the whole organism with vitality. In an unhealthy state, an inversion can occur through psychological conditioning, shock, and trauma, where we lack tonus and have areas of habitual tension. Because of our "tube within tube" formation, when one or more sphincters are held closed, movement is constrained—like holding a finger on a straw—and the fluid cannot move. In this way, any suction in the mouth or chronic tension at the anus, urethra, or any of the sphincter muscles inhibits the movements of peristalsis and digestion, breathing, fluid circulation, and even the quality of voice, etc. We need to free the movement at our core to re-enliven the tonus on our surface.

If you are ready to incorporate this practice into the LUV sequence, I recommend adding it when you reach the first U position … to loosen up any residual tension in the muscles of the back, neck, and limbs. You can also utilize it in this way immediately after any other inversion, to release any residue of tension and help your organism integrate any physiological and structural changes that may have occurred while practicing. However, it is equally valuable to use this "soft-bellied shimmy shake" as a warm-up before such challenging practices as inversions and backbends to prepare yourself to move with ease rather than pushing through by tensing toward an accomplishment.

Practice:

Imagine stroking the soft belly of a kitty, splayed out on your lap, purring in delight. Now imagine you are the kitty. With your arms and legs gently extended in the air, relax your limbs, letting your knees and elbows be loose. Shimmy, keeping the belly soft and freeing the breathing, to a gentle quiver or laugh. Be careful not to hyperventilate or pant. You may find this tiring at first, but try building up slowly from one to three minutes, exploring how much you can relax into the shimmy.

This practice will flush the lymph system, enhancing immune functions, digestion, and endocrine functions, and will bring a new aliveness and tonus while reducing chronic tensions and the overall level of tonic contractions. This disorganizing movement liberates the breathing from habitual patterns that are anchored in the surface skeletal muscles.

Further Differentiations

Straight-leg rise

When you can bring your legs effortlessly into the "L" position from the bent-knee position, then you are ready to experiment with letting your legs rise up straight like spokes of a wheel from the center of your pelvis. As you begin the LUV sequence lying supine, pool the energy of your lower back deeper and deeper into the ground, rather than initiating the rise from the tensing of surface skeletal muscles. On the exhalation, bring the legs up to be perpendicular to the ground, as you pour your lower back ever more deeply.

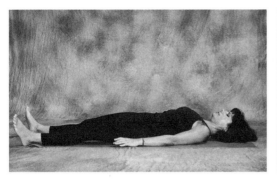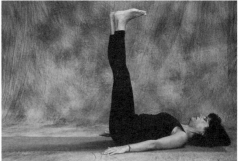

Completing the LUV sequence

Straight-leg return

At the end of the LUV sequence, before you begin your legs' descent to the ground, you can lower your straight legs slowly from the "L" position, reorganizing the structure as you go by deepening the pool of the lower back into the ground. This will allow you to shape-shift, reforming your relationship to ground, so that you can receive the support coming up through your structure the whole way down, rather than controlling the legs by straining your surface skeletal muscles.

The emphasis of this Somatic Meditation is on self-organizing through one's structure and utilizing that as a way of moving in space by simply inviting space and gravity to reshape us. This shape-shifting practice is very different than, for instance, moving one's legs as "objects in space." Pilates and other disciplines utilize exercises that may appear similar in order to develop core strength. The movement of the legs is controlled by holding the abdominal muscles in contraction. While this proves valuable in mitigating back strain, it also proves constraining to the capacity of the organism to fluidly self-organize.

Rest and gravity-reference scan

As you rest do not abandon yourself and leave "the body," letting the mind drift away. With each breath, extend your presence to savor the taste of the infinite as it enters you, opens you. Kiss back to the beloved as you extend your presence on your exhalation. There is no receiving without interpenetration. There is no extending without interpenetration. Everything converges. Every breath is a kissing back.

When you are bathed to your heart's content, having immersed yourself in the infinite substance and dissolved completely, you can rise up. Not as the "object self" to return to the world and its "drying out," but as the unbounded being you have re-membered yourself to be. Let that infinite being rise up and receive the world.

Through these practices, you have entered the fluid world, given up your identifications, and reclaimed your cosmic nature. You have disenthralled from your "image form" to know yourself as unfolding movement, embracing ever-greater freedom and aliveness. You can return to the world and its drying out as a fluid being, rising up, walking on land, retaining the energy of water, learning to live in the world without identifying with the object/image-level consensual reality.

Implications

Having discovered a fluid, non-mechanical way of moving, allow your interest to notice how long this new way of being sustains itself. Notice when the "object body" memory takes over, reasserting itself through habit. This state-shifting can happen very quickly. Finding yourself when you lose yourself necessitates that you notice when you are dropping out—as when you have been reading for a while, and you suddenly notice that you do not remember what you've read in the previous paragraphs. To reclaim yourself from the mechanical activity, you must first notice that you dropped out or disassociated.

As you enter your day from your morning practice, notice when you have left a process-level awareness, or self-sensing, and find yourself back to the fragmentation of I as object. In relationship, for instance, when we are oriented primarily from this fragmented sense of self, we hear one another only through our images of self and other. If we can learn to notice this, we can re-extend our presence. Through this extension of presence, we rediscover and redefine what we take as personal—that which is most immediate and deeply felt—which is, paradoxically, what most deeply connects us to one another.

I offer the following examples to provide a spectrum of ways to play with this through the varied activities of your day.

Brushing your teeth

When you brush your teeth, how much do you tense your shoulder, neck, and facial muscles? What does it feel like when you relax the "efforting"? How much effort do you need to brush your teeth? Are you interested in finding out?

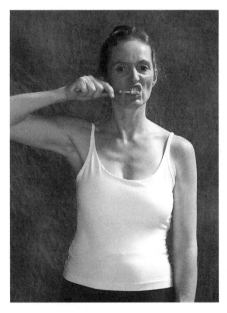 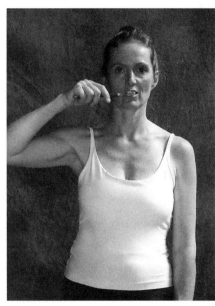

With unnecessary tension   With minimal tension

Seeing yourself in the mirror

Notice if your facial muscles tighten or adjust when you first see your face in the mirror. Close your eyes, empty your breath completely, and as you relax the diaphragms of exhalation, and the breath effortlessly flows to you, also relax any tension you feel in your face. Not a camera smile from the outside in, but a releasing from the inside out. Let that smiling soften your shoulders and melt your arms and back, expressing the warm glow of appreciation and joy. Slowly open your eyes and allow the light to enter through your open lids without grasping the image with your eyes. Feel your presence filling the image in the mirror. Can you see the image without becoming self-conscious? Feel free to play with closing your eyes and opening them as many times as you like, to "refresh" your connection to your here-now, all at once, somatic experiencing and to disenthrall from your identification with the image you see.

Relaxing the sphincters

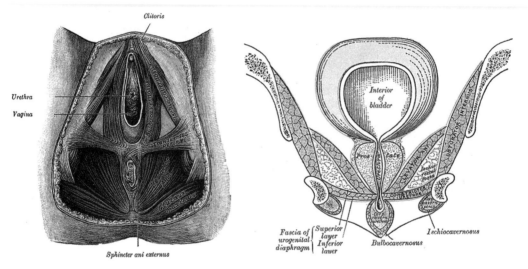

The pelvic sphincters, female and male

Urinary sphincter: When you pee, are you exerting any extra pressure to push the urine out? What happens if you stop the doing? Can you still pee, simply by relaxing your urinary sphincter muscle? How much do you need to relax for the peeing to start? What happens when you empty your bladder completely? Does this muscle remain relaxed? I invite you to check in throughout the day, and explore how much you can let go of this sphincter muscle.

Oral sphincter: Notice when there is a slight suction in your mouth. Just as lifting a straw from a glass of water with your finger enclosing the top will form a suction that holds the water in place, sealing the upper palate of your mouth with your tongue can form a similar suction. It doesn't take much pressure at all to impede the gentle waves of peristalsis or breathing. The effects of this impedance can be quite pervasive, affecting all systems—nervous, digestive, immune, circulatory, endocrine, and so on—to say nothing of your psychology. The more you constrain the mobility and motility of your organs, the less you can feel.

Anal sphincter: Our organization as tubes within tubes, creating a suction at either end or at sphincters midway, can affect the functioning of the whole system. One of the first things we learn as young children is to avert shame. We can create a private world simply by closing down the opening of our mouth or anus. And if we hold both ends tense, we can barely feel anything until we relax our holding. In this way we learn to gain some control over our own experience, thereby insulating us from the harsh humiliations of life. But at what cost?

Sense how much more transparent you are when you let go of these holdings. Each time you check in again, are they back? Is it safe for you to let in all that you feel? Can you self-soothe when you need comfort and ease without judgment?

Talking on the phone

When you talk on the telephone, how forcefully do you grip the handset? What muscles are involved in the gripping? Your neck, shoulders, arm, hand? Can you relax your grip? If you find this difficult, start by exaggerating the tensing you are doing, incrementally. Once you learn how you are doing this, it is easier to release what you actually are doing, rather than making compensations for it.

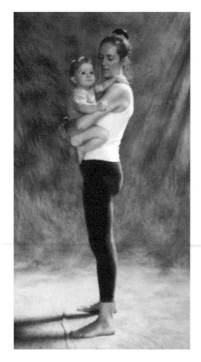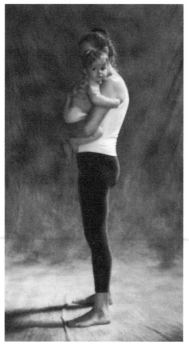

With strain   Embracing to relax the holding

Carrying a baby (or a heavy object)—
Gravity as adversary, gravity as ally

How much straining is going on when you carry your baby? Can you relax your holding and let the baby's weight pour through your fluid structure, sinking like a stone in water? Let gravity have its way with you, shape-shifting your structure as it draws the weight into the earth. Let gravity deliver you from any tension. Let the Earth carry the weight, not your muscles. If you stop carrying the baby as a weight in your arms, you can begin sensing your interrelationship as a "convergence of rivers." Does embracing your baby in this way enhance your enjoyment?

Driving

How much do you "push" your car down the street when you drive? Can you enjoy the ride even when you are late? Does it help you to stay connected to where you think you should be by not enjoying the present where you are? Do you get there any faster by tensing up? Since you have to sit there anyway, why not gravity-surf as you drive? As the breath comes to you, release any tension you feel to receive the breath at your depths. When you exhale, ride the omnidirectional wave through your structure and beyond. How does it feel when you stop tensing toward the destination and let the road come to you? Does your driving become smoother? Do you find yourself more present when you arrive?

Coquelicot, one of the practitioners in my training program, drove many hours to get to each training. At first the drives felt like a burden, and she arrived tired and stressed. When she realized that she could take the long drive as uninterrupted time to deepen her practice of Somatic Learning, she leapt at the opportunity. She began arriving very refreshed, almost blissfully happy.

Tatiana's Story: Transforming Limitations and "Pain" by Stopping the "Trying"

A beautiful and talented clothes designer and performance artist had suffered for years from chronic fatigue that she found debilitating. She was in so much pain and so weak that she was barely walking. When she moved to the U.S. in her thirties, she remembers having to use a wheelchair just to get through the airports.

I had been ill for some time and had not made any improvement. Somatic Learning was not trying to improve my physical body or its story, but rather to lead me into a direct identification with spirit—the non-visible source within me. I learned so much more than I had thought possible. I realized that the problems came from over-identifying with a physical body and its story, and that the answer to my problems was not outside me.

Some of the benefits I began to experience included an increased ability to relax and feel connected internally. Through the invitation to practice minute attention, micro-movement, and non-spatial movement, I could transform limitations and pain by stopping the "trying" and "doing." I began letting go and relaxing. I developed a loving, working relationship with gravity, beauty, and physical grace. I stopped hitting the body against a physical world, and no longer lugged the physical body around like a disabled burden. I reclaimed height and good posture; my spine grew one and three-quarters inches in the first two years of practice (in my forties). I also have a sense of self-forgiveness as a result of decompressing my vertebrae, which had become nearly fused together through calcification from all the compression.

What gave me relief was the confidence developed by creating space where I didn't think I could, and the ability to dissolve lifelong stress and pain. I gave up drama, competition, effort, and ambition.

Because I was able to dissolve pain, I was more comfortable in my physical body and therefore less angry and reactive to others. My ability to relate kindly and intimately with other people grew. I was able to sustain a pregnancy (after five miscarriages) and to willingly transform fear, burden, and shame.

The biggest change that occurred was through maintaining a daily practice of Somatic Learning: that was what supported me in sustaining these transformative changes without the need for a teacher as an outside authority.

Developing my practice is more fun than the old way of trying to perfect it. In this sense, it feels like the main blockage to practice might simply be ambition.

I also discovered how key the sacrum is—the more I find it, the more I experience it, not only as the key but also as the door that allows tumbling into the unknown: just as Alice changed her shape enough to fit through the door into Wonderland. It is often simpler than I expect. For instance, the sacrum is already shaped like an arrow, already pointing in the direction it wants to take me. If I let it follow that direction, the rest unfolds on its own. What a different experience it is from trying to make perfect shapes with my body, and then as a teacher instructing others to do the same. As a student, as a teacher, the falling through becomes easier the more I practice.

The overall impact on my life was developing the ability to go through whatever is calling and pass through it to the natural peace beyond it. I constantly rededicate myself to choose peace instead of settling for drama, competition, and fear. I've begun to see the world as a state of mind rather than a place. Every moment I recognize that, I recognize that I have the power to change it.

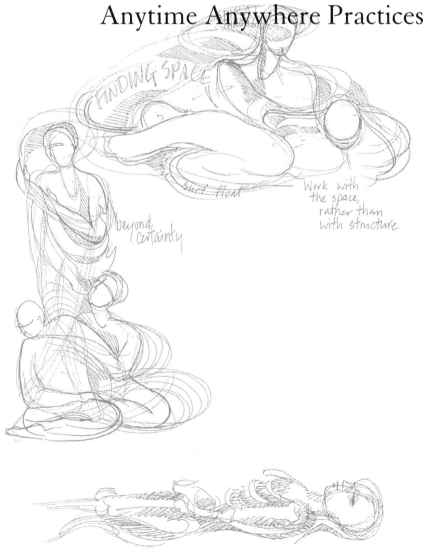

PART III

The Art and Practice of Somatic Learning: Anytime Anywhere Practices

FINDING SPACE

surf float

Work with
the space,
rather than
with structure

beyond
certainty

Through the sea of soft tissue I call my body
liquid landscapes pulsing
I sense the heartbeat
  this blue planet
The vigorous yes green
Longing itself
  toward light.
Here where rolling water
and upright water meet
where I call home.

—*Risa Kaparo, from the poem "Living On Island"*[1]

CHAPTER 9

Anytime Anywhere Practices: Standing

These Anytime Anywhere Practices are an opportunity to carry your practice "beyond the mat" and to integrate your awakened somatic intelligence throughout the day.

If you began your morning with the Bedtime or Morning practices, you are entering your day from a more dimensionally extended presence. However, especially in the beginning, more than likely this extended presence will diminish—either gradually or when something suddenly triggers old programming.

How aware you are of the feedback your organism provides determines how far down the line you notice symptoms developing. Perhaps you may start to move more mechanically or less efficiently as habitual tensions reemerge; eventually even chronic pain may reappear.

As with your car, are you aware of the gas gauge dipping, or do you wait until the warning light comes on … or finally notice when the car chugs to a stop? Research on chronic pain reveals the influence of feedback. This calls to mind a study I remember reading many years ago, which I am including to vivify the power of feedback, though I can no longer find that particular study to reference it exactly. In the study, participants with chronic back pain were given belts to wear, attached to sensors that were placed on the surface skeletal muscles of their back When these muscles began to contract, a yellow light went on in the belt. When the muscles were in the state of high tension, a red light came on. The researchers intended to monitor the participants for three months to see how the feedback affected the chronic pain; however, the study ended early because after three weeks, there was no more chronic pain to monitor.

Just as Tibetan Buddhist meditation instruction points out, you can either catch the movement of thought at the head … or way down the line at the tail end, after being dragged around by it for some time without awareness.

As the previously presented Arthurian fairytale about Lady Ragnell illustrates (see Chapter 4), no matter how transformative the initial insight into another mode of experiencing, it doesn't hold indefinitely under all circumstances. We keep changing from the beautiful young maiden to the old hag. This is the very reason for having a practice: to reawaken ever more quickly when you fall out and regress into a less differentiated functioning. Without awareness you cannot reclaim yourself from the old programs that operate subconsciously, running you ragged.

When you recognize that you have lost your connection, what follows is most critical. Either shame will turn the insight against you, perpetuating the story of not good enough, or interest will follow, reconnecting you to what actually sustains you. I am most grateful to my practice, because at any time, even when shame scripts get the best of me, connection is no more than a breath away. The breath has become for me the embrace that dispels the curse … at once revealing beauty and renewing me.

Practice is how we dispel the reemergence of the curse. When something inevitably triggers old programs and beliefs that reshape your biology, know that this is a gift. At that moment the infrastructure of your thought system reveals itself. You get to see the old programming that is still operable under those particular circumstances.

Another principle from Buddhist practice is KIKI, often translated as "crisis." The word "crisis" in Japanese *(kiki)* has the kanji (character) for "danger" and the kanji for "opportunity." When we recognize what is happening as an opportunity and embrace it, alert to the dangers without becoming paralyzed by fear, we are ripe for transformative learning and change. Feeling both the urgency and the gravity of a situation provides the dual necessities that render us ripe. As Krishnamurti often said, "You must feel your house burning." If you don't sense the urgency, you do not find the requisite energy to change your life. At the same time, if you just react to the sense of urgency without letting it turn to gravity within you, you will merely perpetuate the problem by reacting from the same conditions from which the problem arose.

We must feel the urgency but not react to it from our old programming. When we let the gravity of a situation move through us, what comes to ground in us is a newly awakened response-ability.

For example, when I teach Somatic Learning touchwork to practitioners, I begin with Somatic Meditations involving what are generally experienced as relatively fixed, inanimate objects. When the practitioners' touch can interpenetrate with these "objects" (wood blocks, rocks, etc.) like rivers converging, they are ready to move on to working with other humans. One such experiment involves holding a rock in hand. Holding its weight eventually reveals our tensional patterns—how we habitually hold ourselves in an adversarial relationship to gravity. If we stop resisting gravity and begin to sense how gravity draws the weight of the rock toward the center of the Earth, and we get out of its way by releasing the old tensions that this awareness reveals, we allow gravity to liberate us.

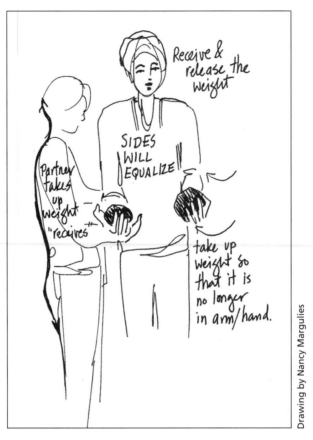

Receive & release the weight

SIDES WILL EQUALIZE

Partner takes up weight "receives"

take up weight so that it is no longer in arm/hand.

Drawing by Nancy Margulies

Equalizing weight with rocks in hand

Transforming Your Relationship to Gravity

Gravity delivers us when we stop fighting it. When we receive it as gift. It is in the receiving, in the embrace, that the curse is dispelled and transformation occurs.

The heart of Somatic Learning practice is this embrace, this orientation to receive *what is* as gift. Practice leads to confidence. This confidence grows faith, a general orientation of gratefulness. As discussed earlier, nature reveals itself to us according to how we probe. Quantum mechanics has articulated this as the principle of non-determinacy. Remember the example of light revealing itself as a wave or a particle according to how we probe it. Through gratefulness—this orientation to receive what is as gift—we are poised to invent/discover a gift in whatever occurs. When you move through life with the spirit of gratefulness as your general orientation, the world reveals itself to you as grace.

ELLEN'S STORY: BECOMING LIGHTNESS, EASE, AND COMFORT

Ellen, a journalist in her thirties, came to the work suffering from a severe scoliosis that twisted her spine like a corkscrew. The extent to which her spine realigned from her experiences with Somatic Learning and related disciplines thoroughly surprised her. She has continued to shed density, to live pain-free and move with increasing ease and grace since she began her practice a quarter-century ago.

I recently had a dream about my embodied self of some twenty-five years ago. In the dream, the younger person I was sits in a small amphitheater-style classroom. What is striking is the image of me twisted from head to toe, shoulders and torso rotated, the torque not just in the spine but embedded in the surprisingly heavy density of the body. I felt I had been given a view into the past to mark what I've become in terms of lightness, ease, and comfort.

My work with Dr. Kaparo began serendipitously many years ago with her first yoga class after she returned from intensive study with master Vanda Scaravelli. Yoga had always been a way that I could feel at home in myself. But this Somatic Learning class was different in that its focus would eventually lead to a universe of ideas and a heightened capacity to experience life as a function of attention. The Somatic Meditations have been a way to literally "press" life into my being through attention in an immediate way. I recognize this capacity in the way a jazz singer may begin a song—without a hair's breadth of hesitation or self-consciousness. One moment no sound, and then in the next we are fully taken up into the immediacy of the music. This work is a kind of salvation.

Gravity-Reference Scan (Standing)

As in the Bedtime and Morning practices, doing a gravity-reference scan (this time from standing) provides an opportunity to embrace "what is," to remember who you truly are: infinite consciousness embodied in an energy form. You want to begin from this embrace, from beauty (as Vanda would say), rather than from an orientation of trying to fix something. "Trying" is the operative word, because whatever you do to adjust yourself mechanically will only create more complex patterns of compensation that will lead you on a wild goose chase of "doing." Before you know it, you are at the tail end of having chased an image.

The gravity-reference scan provides you with a physical reference (starting baseline) so that you can more easily and accurately assess any changes that might occur with your practice.

Duration: One minute or longer
Instructions

Stand in a relaxed position without trying to impose an image of good posture. We want to find out what muscles are still "working" when we are at rest. There are no right or wrong answers.

Questions/Inquiries to reflect on

- Notice any areas of pain or discomfort.
- Sense your weight distribution—notice what percentage of your weight falls on the left versus right leg.
- How much weight falls on the ball of the foot versus on the heel?
- Do your toes curl or grasp?
- How much weight falls on the outside edge versus the inside edge of the foot?
- Is one shoulder higher than the other?
- What is the angle of your head? For example, is your head leaning forward or is your chin out, in, up, or down?

- How pronounced are the curvatures of the spine? Is the curve of your upper back exaggerated and bending you forward (kyphosis)? Or is the curve of your lower back exaggerated and hyper-extended (lordosis)?
- What parts of your structure feel heavy or hard to hold up?
- What parts of your structure feel light?
- What parts of your structure feel hardly present or externally related (e.g., your arms)?
- What parts feel relatively fixed and what parts feel more flowing?
- Where do you feel direct support from the ground? In your feet, through your legs? In your pelvis, lower back, upper back, neck, or head?
- What is supporting your head?
- Can you feel the support of the ground through your skeleton, or do you rely on the muscles of your neck to hold your head upright?
- Where do you sense your muscles tensing to hold yourself up? In your neck, in your upper or lower back, in your thighs, calves, ankles, your shoulders?
- What structures move when you breathe? Your belly? Which ribs? Back or front? Do you sense any movement in your legs or arms or head?
- Observe your observing—how do you watch, how does your attention operate?
- Does your attention operate like a flashlight, shining from point to point?
- Is the process of paying attention changing the way you are?
- Now make a mental picture of your posture (i.e., the alignment of your structure) and whatever you discovered, so later you can notice changes that occur.

Implications

All your observations are assets when it comes to knowing what has changed when you experiment with the upcoming exercises.

Differentiation is one of the core processes that inform your Somatic Learning. Again, by "differentiation" we mean the ability to notice increasingly subtle changes or movements. The more we sense differences, the more responsive we are and more efficient our movements become. When we are not adding extra tension, we are more sensitive.

You may notice that certain things begin to change from "just observing" them. How interesting!

Finding Neutral (Standing Position)

Standard Weight-Shifting Reference

Side-to-side axis

1. Start by shifting your weight to the left as you ordinarily would (putting more weight on one leg and on the edges of your feet). Return to center and repeat this several times.
2. Now shift your weight to the right (putting more weight on one leg) and return to center. Repeat.

Front-to-back axis

1. Shift your weight forward (putting more weight on the balls of the feet). Notice if your toes start gripping the ground, or if your legs and back stiffen. Return to center and repeat several times to sense what happens in your structure as you move.
2. Try shifting your weight backward (putting more weight on the heels). Come back to center and repeat.

Observations

When you shifted your weight to the right or left, did you notice your hip go out to the side and your torso compensate by leaning to the opposite

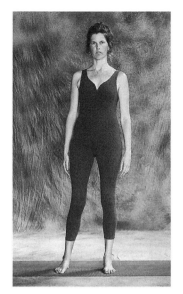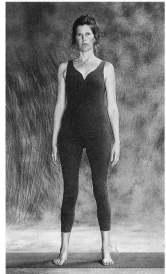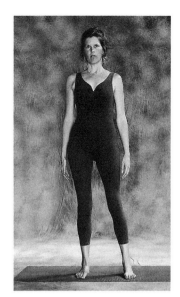

Shifting weight to determine neutral position

side? Likewise, when you shifted your weight forward and back, did you notice your muscles gripping your own skeleton as well as the ground (with your toes). This is what I refer to as "compensational adjustment." The "object body" moves mechanically to compensate as you change your relationship to the gravitational field, as though the parts of the body were relatively fixed and externally related like the limbs of a doll.

Now let's experiment with a non-mechanical mode of sensing and initiating movement.

Somatic Learning Weight-Shifting

Side-to-side axis

1. Receive the ground through the left side, drinking it up as though you were a tree drinking in the moisture through your roots, drawing it up the trunk of your legs and torso, and out the branches of your head and arms to nourish the leaves.

2. Now do the same through the right side. Allow this drinking to shift where your weight is supported, without moving your body

mechanically. Instead of your weight shifting from above, your weight remains rooted in the ground (where it belongs) as the support rises through the other leg.

3. See how effortlessly and fluidly your structure can shape-shift as you repeat this weight shift several times. Now find your neutral standing position by relaxing all your muscles. Sense how your weight is supported in the ground.

4. Notice the difference in shifting your weight mechanically from above the ground (the first way) and how you feel when you shift your weight with somatic awareness (non-mechanically) from below, through the convergence of your organism and the ground.

Front-to-back axis

1. Receive the support of the ground now through the balls of your feet, without shifting your weight from above. When the shift in support happens from below, there will not be a stiffening of your muscles against your skeleton or any gripping the ground with your toes. Keep the motion small to sense the subtle self-organizing throughout your structure, not just in your feet and ankles.

2. Receive the support of the ground now through your heels, sensing how your structure shape-shifts as it receives the support of the ground rising up through your torso, head, and arms.

3. Repeat the process several times to see how smoothly and gradually you can flow forward and back to center. Now relax all your muscles and see how your weight is supported from the ground.

Observations

You may have noticed that when your weight is held "above ground" your balance is much more precarious. When your weight is held inside the ground like a tree, you don't lose balance because you are "rooted."

The Art and Practice of Somatic Learning: Anytime Anywhere Practices

You find support without needing to rely on muscular tension to gird your structure upright. When the support comes from the ground up, you needn't keep making minute adjustments to maintain balance, because you are no longer holding yourself up.

You have transformed your relationship to gravity. Gravity becomes your ally rather than adversary.

Unlike a fixed object, such as the doll mentioned earlier, all your "parts" are intrinsically related to the whole and capable of changing shape. Instead of mechanically adjusting yourself to compensate for your changing relationship to the gravitational field, you begin to shape-shift fluidly. Rather than relating to yourself from the outside, as an observer (which perpetuates the image/object-level orientation), your somatic intelligence is self-sensing, self-organizing, and self-renewing.

Whatever aspects of this transformation you have experienced at this point will serve you as a portal into a realm of greater freedom and aliveness. You needn't feel concerned if you have not embodied these insights completely. As you continue with your practice, you will develop ever more subtle levels of differentiation and learn to extend your presence beyond the limitations of the known, opening infinitely. Give importance to whatever you experience, even when it is different from the observations that I have described. We enter the realm of endless possibilities by embracing "what is" here-now, which will keep changing with every breath.

> People are going back and forth across the doorsill
> where the two worlds touch. The door is round and open.
> Don't go back to sleep!
> —*Rumi*

You will inevitably go back and forth across the portal where the two worlds meet (i.e., the consensual realm of "object-level" awareness and the dimensionally extended realm of somatic intelligence). This is the practice of self-mastery. Find yourself again and again by re-extending your presence through somatic awareness.

Implications

Since the mechanical way of moving the "body as object" is based on an image or inferential way of knowing yourself, it requires ongoing effort to maintain upright posture through endless compensations.

Relying on visual perception (observation from the "mind's eye" searching out ground—a long way down there somewhere) from a point of observation in the head freezes the position of the head so that it no longer responds to the ground. It not only proves inadequate to rely on visual perception where proprioception is needed, this "synesthesia"[2] (replacing or confusing one sense perception for another) perpetuates your dissociation from the ground and gravitational field. From this dissociated state of consciousness, you experience yourself as separate and needing to fight an endless war with gravity to maintain your upright position. Some researchers have estimated that eighty percent of our brain functioning is occupied in this struggle to hold ourselves up, to say nothing of all the muscular wear and tear that is both unnecessary and actually constraining to our freedom and aliveness.

Somatic awareness, the "all at once, here-now mode of perception," dispels the curse of this identification as a dissociated self, experienced as a separate object mechanically locomoting through space.

Remember not to rush through this exploration, tensing toward an accomplishment. There is no "there" to get to. Our ambition comes from imposing our images or ideals on "what is." As Vanda Scaravelli reminded her students: "Infinite time, no ambition. No ambition, infinite time." If we move too quickly through this exploration, we will miss the implications, trying to get somewhere. As Brother David Steindl-Rast describes: "Leisure is not the privilege of those who can afford to take time, it is the virtue of those who give to everything they do the time it deserves to take." The practice is not for accomplishment, but awakening.

Calling through the Horizon from Standing Position

Receiving through the Eyes

Duration: Two minutes

Intention

To feel greater freedom and aliveness by inviting more space into our structure.

Instructions

Look through a window with an open view of the horizon. Or you can just imagine the horizon in front of you as far as you can see. Imagine the horizon coming to you, through your eyes and through the back of your head. Let the horizon in front of you connect with the horizon behind you. Keep your gaze relaxed, without trying to focus your eyes on anything. The eyes act as a lens, but the seeing is occurring from the visual cortex, at the back of the head.

If you are finding this a challenge, try it with your eyes closed. Now open your eyes slowly as though you were opening the shutters on a camera and just letting in the light.

How can you assess your practice? If you measure yourself against an image of how you think you should look from the outside, you will start compensationally adjusting and thereby perpetuate the violence inherent in this disassociated orientation. It will prove more valuable to sense from the inside.

Do you feel greater freedom, e.g., does the head feel less fixed or held? Do you feel greater aliveness, e.g., more energy, more flow, more connection? You may feel like your head is floating—like a bobble-head doll. You might even notice a change in the position of your head without trying to adjust it muscularly.

Receiving through the Navel

Bring the horizon through your center—just below your navel and out the other side.

Try cupping a hand and placing it on your lower back. Sense the energy overflowing your hand. Now remove your hand but keep sensing the energy flowing through—you can invent an imaginary partner that helps you, and their support can be as real as your imagination is vivid. Another way to think of this exercise is to imagine an ocean in front of you, and you are drawing it through your navel, as if drinking it in through a straw.

Assessing your practice

Do you feel greater freedom, e.g., does the sacrum gently release when you bring the horizon through your center? Do you feel greater aliveness? You may feel like your pelvis is floating on top of your legs.

You might even notice a change in the curvature of your spine or less tension in your legs, back, neck, shoulders.

Receiving through the Heart

Drink in the horizon from as far as you can imagine behind you as it enters through your thoracic spine (at the level of your ribs) and overflows through your heart and lungs, pouring out your chest wall and kissing back the infinite. Savor the spaciousness you presence by sensing the omni-directional convergence of inexhaustible emptiness and luminosity in embodied mindfulness.

Restoring Natural Breathing (Standing)

(For a complete review of Somatic Learning breathing, please refer to Chapter 6.)

Duration: Two minutes

Intention

Since the only way to substantially deepen your breathing is to employ the diaphragms of exhalation, the more completely we empty our lungs, the more completely we fill them. This practice restores us to our natural, deep breathing.

Have you ever watched a baby breathe? You can see every part of her moving on the waves of her breath. Unfortunately, this natural movement diminishes as we age and habitually rely on muscles to hold ourselves up.

Practice suggestion

Begin with Finding Neutral (Standing Position) and Calling through the Horizon practices.

Instructions

Leave the mouth closed with the jaw relaxed. Imagine for a moment that you have a bellows extending from the floor of your pelvis to the base of your skull.

Exhalation: Now empty the bellows without tensing the muscles of your back, especially activating the pelvic diaphragm at the floor of the pelvis. Do not strain to push all the air out using pressure—just let the bellows empty as fully as possible without straining.

Inhalation: Slowly relax and feel how the bellows fills up with air on its own—without straining to suck air in through your nostrils. Gradually relax the diaphragms and any muscular tension that you find to receive the breath more fully. Repeat several times, emptying the bellows and letting the breath come to you without effort.

Now place your hands over your kidneys at the base of your rib cage in back. As you exhale follow the movement of the bellows closing with your hands, emptying out from your sides at the level of your kidneys. Again, when you come to be empty, relax and slowly let the breath come to you. Do this several times until you feel your lungs empty smoothly and gently from the base all the way to the top.

Now sense both the vertical and horizontal flows to feel yourself rhythmically emptying from all directions as the diaphragms gently embrace your core and release, effortlessly filling out in all directions. Allow the exhalation to be more active and the inhalation to be more passive.

Assessing your practice

Do you feel more freedom and aliveness, e.g., is your breathing fuller or deeper? Does more of your structure move with your breath? Do you feel more relaxed and more alert at the same time? Is your mind quieting down?

Quick Spinal Release (Standing)

This is a version of the spinal elongation that utilizes the flexing of the knees to amplify the omnidirectional wave going through the spine. It is basically the same movement as the quick spinal release from lying in Chapter 7, "Bedtime Practices"—except that the position offers a different relationship to gravity. We will anchor the wave through the arms as well.

Quick reference: Take a moment to bend your knees slightly as you regularly would to gain a baseline for later comparison. As always, make sure you do not strain yourself. Do not overdo. (Bigger is not better!)

Notice: Where does your weight fall in your foot? How much weight is in your knees? Does your body go down when you bend and up when you straighten your knees?

Instructions

From a neutral standing position, imagine that you are being held up from a string attached to the top of your head that does not let your head go down as your knees bend. Your spine will elongate to make the extra space needed to bend the knees.

Exhaling: Initiate the emptying from the pelvic floor. (See instructions for "Restoring Natural Breathing [Standing]" on page 218.) As the sacrum anchors, slowly soften the knees so they bend naturally, but only slightly.

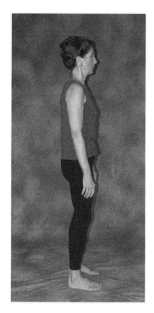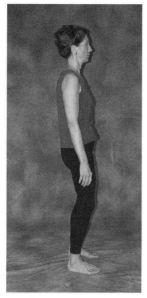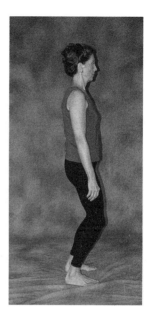

Quick spinal release in standing position

By "anchoring," I mean extending your presence beyond your structure as you sense gravity pull you toward the center of the Earth. Sense the anchors as portals, opening you to an immediately apprehensible felt-sense of your connection to both heaven and earth, and all that is.

Notice that your weight does not go into your knees—but transfers through them and goes down through your heels.

Inhaling: Relax everything completely and sense the breath coming to you as you relax your diaphragms (let the bellows open on its own) and rest with your knees slightly bent.

Exhaling: Now slowly extend (straighten) your knees while you sense the force of gravity anchoring you. Even though these instructions are given sequentially, you are to practice them all at once (simultaneously). Initially, you can try one quick spinal release (through a sequence of two exhalations and two inhalations, which constitutes one knee bend since you are bending and extending the knee on one exhalation each). Focus on each of the anchors to ground them.

Anchoring of your sacrum—amplifying the wave up the spine: The anchoring of the sacrum will pull the lower two lumbar vertebrae downward, while the upper two lumbar vertebrae will ride the wave releasing the spine upward. Thus, the center of the omnidirectional wave occurs around the waistline. Anchor the base of your skull (occiput and jaw)— amplifying the wave up through the head. Rather than the head bobbing like one ball over the spine, find the subtle anchor of the skull, engendering movement throughout the cranium. Thus the twenty-two bones of the face and skull can gently open like the petals of a lotus flower.

Anchor through your heels—amplifying the wave through the legs and the base of the spine: This enables us as bipeds to enjoy a connection to the ground through our spine, similar to quadrupeds. All twenty-eight bones of the feet elongate and root into the ground like a tree. The heel sends a large taproot, while the other bones grow a finer lace of roots, deeper and deeper into the earth.

Inhaling: Relax everything completely and sense the breath coming to you as you relax your diaphragms—let the bellows open on their own.

Now sense the omnidirectional wave through the spine as a whole, while you repeat the quick spinal release. While the primary wave moves vertically, from the waist down and from the waist up, you can sense the convergence of these waves moving omnidirectionally through all parts.

Opening the crown: Repeat the knee bend on your next breath—this time anchoring through your jaw and the base of your skull.

Assess your practice

At this point, you may feel your spine elongating in both the bending and extending of your knees.

Do you feel more freedom and aliveness? Generally when our knees are bent, our lower back relaxes and extends. With this practice we learn how to elongate the spine, so that even in an extended knee position the lower back remains open.

Note: This is essentially the same as the quick spinal release from supine position that appeared in the Bedtime practices. The difference is the change in your relationship to the gravitational field from lying to standing.

The practice vivifies the reciprocal relationship between your knees and lower back. If your lower back remains open, the knees cannot lock no matter how much you extend them. Conversely, if you compress your lower back, your knees will lock or bear weight. This is why anchoring down from your sacrum is so important. It holds your lower back open.

Variation: Using Weights

Instructions

Placing a light weight (1–3 lbs.) in each hand, repeat the elongation. The weight can vivify the anchoring through the hands, to help you sense the elongation along the entire length of the arm. If you have ever seen a salt-water taffy machine, you may remember how the weight at the bottom lengthens the taffy.

Now without the weights, repeat the elongation, imagining invisible weights in your hands.

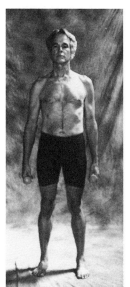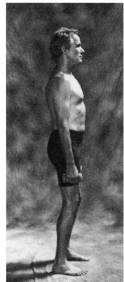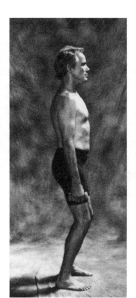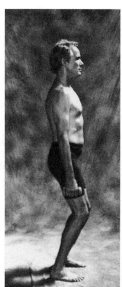

Sensing the elongation using weights

Variation: Partner Facilitation

If you have a partner to work with, the facilitator can support you in sensing the wave of elongation more vividly by sending energy down through the anchors listed above.

Without a partner, you can self-facilitate with your own touch, utilizing the following touch-points to amplify your sensing of gravity and the wave of the intrinsic movement.

1. Placing one hand just below the navel and the other across from it at the back of the spine, feel the "energy" flow through your hands as (you or) your partner brings through the horizon.
2. Placing a hand on the base of the skull and one hand on the forehead, feel the head float when your partner brings through the horizon.
3. Place one hand on the sacrum and one hand on the thoracic spine, as shown in the photo. While you elongate, you can best support your partner in anchoring through the sacrum and receiving the wave up through the thoracic spine, creating more space between

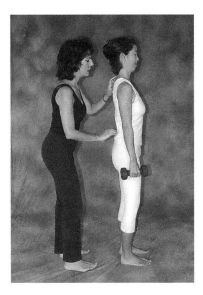

Quick spinal release with partner facilitation

the vertebrae that lie between your hands. If you are practicing self-facilitation, feel free to modify this one to touch your sternum with one hand and your sacrum with the other.

Assessing your practice

Any of the following sensations will indicate that you are releasing and extending your spine:

- Your neck elongates as the pressure of the head is released.
- Your skull expands.
- Your jaw relaxes.
- Your ears and eyes open and come more alive—almost as if someone turned a monitor on.

Opening the Heart

The arms serve as an anchor to hold open the portal of the heart that you opened when drinking in the horizon. You will extend your presence along the horizontal dimension now, carrying or expressing into the world (through your arms) the energy flowing through the heart and central vertical channel (through the spine, head, and legs).

There is a release of energy when the wave moves through the thoracic spine, making space between vertebrae. When you drink in the energy through your arms, the space in the armpits opens, floating the arms freely in space. As you channel it down through the elbows, wrists, and fingers, the energy will flow unobstructed through both the horizontal and vertical channels. The arms will elongate, opening the joints, lengthening the muscles. Thus, the arms will hang more like pendulums rather than at foreshortened angles due to habitual tension.

Without this unobstructed flow, the space between the vertebrae that emerged in the wave of elongation will collapse back in on itself. It is this collapsing of the energy that densifies the structure. When the energy is able to flow unobstructed, the structure sheds its density.

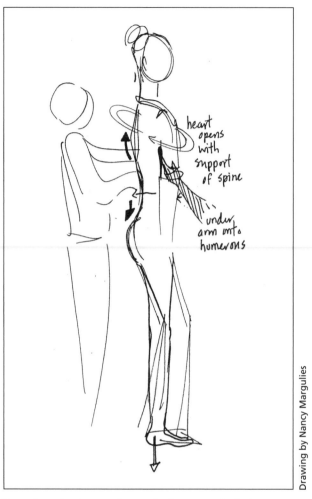

heart opens with support of spine

under arm onto humerous

Drawing by Nancy Margulies

Opening the heart through the portal of the arms

Instructions

Right Arm: On the wave of your next breath, extend your presence through your right arm as described above. As the elongation moves down your arm, maintain the space in the armpit. Savor this for several breaths.

What did you notice as a result of this practice?

Does your right arm feel different than your left? What about the throat? Can you sense a difference between the right and left sides? If you make an open-throated sound like an "A," do you sense a difference in vibration from one side to another? Do your right eye and ear feel more open than your left? Do they feel lit up, like a monitor came on?

Left Arm: Repeat channeling the wave through the left arm. Then integrate both arms.

What did you notice as a result of this practice? Do you feel more openness in your chest? Less density in your upper back? More energy flowing through your arms and hands?

Spinal Elongation (Standing, without Knee Bend)

Duration: Two minutes

Intention

To release strain and density by extending sensing beyond your structure into the larger environment. You will learn to sense the omnidirectional wave that decompresses your spine. You will feel more supported by your skeleton, and less reliant on your muscles for support, freeing them for movement.

Practice suggestions

Begin with Finding Neutral and Calling Through the Horizon practices, as well as Restoring Natural Breathing (all from Standing Position and all previously introduced in this chapter).

Instructions

When you bring the horizon through your center, sense your sacrum anchoring naturally. Exhale using the bellows breathing—and sense even greater freedom for the sacrum to anchor as the pelvic floor diaphragm rises. Remember, by "anchoring," I am referring to how the weight moves through the sacrum, not a movement in space.

With each exhale: Sense the movement of your sacrum from the inside—like an anchor falling through water, relaxing your lower back. Extend your sensing to feel this weight anchoring you to the center of the

Earth, without tensing your muscles. The deeper the anchoring of your sacrum downward, the more vivid the wave coming up your spine will be. Allow your vertebrae to float upward, riding the wave of your exhalation, inviting space between each vertebra. Feel the wave go out the top of your head and continue upward as far as you can extend your presence.

When you feel your weight shift back more through your heels, extend your presence to root into the ground.

Note: The anchoring of your sacrum should occur without tensing the muscles of your buttocks or tucking your pelvis under.

Standing Pour Forward

Duration: Two minutes or as long as you stay interested

Intention

In this practice you learn to pour forward, effortlessly reorganizing your whole structure through elongating your spine. Rather than just stretching the muscles, this elongation opens all the joints, activating the lengthening reflex that extends the actual muscle fibers.

The elongation is made possible by anchoring the sacrum as you further extend through your knees from an already extended position. (Just as in the quick spinal release; however, this time you start from the knees already extended rather than going from bent to extended.) Remember that anchoring the sacrum will prevent the knees from locking. It is important to avoid locking the knees.

Like the quick spinal release and spinal elongation, this practice is initiated from the waist down. The movement from the waist through the head comes as a result of what you do from the waist down.

Practice suggestions

Begin with Quick Spinal Release (Standing) or Spinal Elongation (Standing, without knee bend).

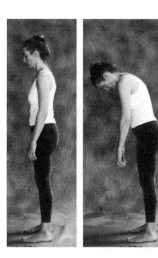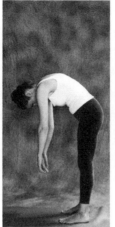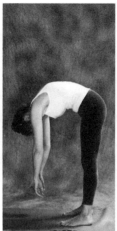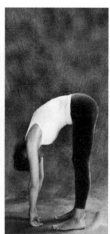

Standing pour forward

Instructions

Stand with feet hip distance apart and parallel. As you inhale, relax and let your weight shift slightly forward toward the balls of the feet.

On the exhalation, simultaneously extend the back of your knees while anchoring the sacrum, to amplify the elongation through your spine. Extend through the knees as though you were a plant yearning for the light. This "yearning" happens without efforting. The plant simply grows toward what it loves most—the beloved sunlight. This growth involves every cell of the plant, from the deepest root through the stems and leaves to the tip of the flowers.

It is also critical that these two anchoring movements (extending the knees and anchoring the sacrum) happen at once. Otherwise you will just go back and forth, rather than changing your structure. Don't be ambitious about going down or strive to touch the ground. In fact, it works better if you "resist" the temptation to reach down, in favor of feeling the wave move through your structure before gravity draws you down. The pouring forward happens as a consequence of this elongation of your spine and gravity, not from anything you do from the waist up.

It is at the end of the elongation, when the wave has moved beyond the top of your head and beyond your feet, that the pour forward begins.

Imagine that warm sunlight is pouring through an open window onto your back and melting you like butter so you pour through a spout at the top of your head.

When you pour water out of a pitcher, all the water moves at the same time. The water at the bottom of the pitcher doesn't wait to move until its turn to go through the spout. It is moving the whole time. Likewise, begin pouring forward from your heels and through the "spout" at the top of your head all at once, as you continue anchoring the movement at the sacrum and the knee.

If you are sensing in a way that is intrinsically connected through the arms, they will feel weightless and relaxed. As the upper part of the spine pours forward at the end of each elongation, the arms float, gently spiraling like two pendulums, with each wave moving through your spine. The movement originates from your spine, not from the arms. If you are not feeling your arms float in this way, you are likely to be tensing through your back and reaching forward with your arms. Or you may not be present in your arms to sense the wave float them. Either way the wave through the spine will be lost to the arms, and they will become an encumbrance.

It is important to continue letting the weight move slightly forward toward the ball of the foot as you relax with each inhale. This keeps your pelvis directly over your feet, avoiding a tendency to move backward, which inhibits the elongation. With each new exhale, ride the omnidirectional wave of elongation through the spine, by extending your knees as you anchor the sacrum.

Stop pouring forward before you experience any strain, so that you are comfortable playing in this position for a more few breaths to see how the elongation deepens there, even without going further down. It doesn't matter how far forward you go, as the practice is about elongating the spine in this relationship to gravity. In fact, if you have elongated well, you can rest in this position comfortably, if you did not fold over in a way that inhibits the belly.

If your hands touch the ground, do not lean your weight forward onto them. Simply rest your palms at the sides of your feet and extend presence into the ground through your hands without pushing. You can also hold the back of your heels, but resist the temptation to pull yourself further down, stretching the surface of your skeletal muscles. Remember this practice is about elongating, not stretching. This necessitates lengthening through the joints and spine, so the soft tissue is obliged to reorganize itself around the new length of your skeleton. This activates the lengthening reflex, physiologically.

Pouring back up to standing

You will come up on an exhalation, initiating the motion by anchoring your sacrum. Think of pulling down on the cord of a curtain rod (to move the curtain). The anchoring of the sacrum functions like a pulley, rooting the energy down into the ground through your legs. This draws the vertebrae up, floating them one above the other as you pour up. Do not tense the muscles of your back or neck to lift your weight. Leave your weight in the ground—where it belongs!

If you sense proprioceptively through your structure as a whole, rather than depending on visual perception to watch and control your "object body," your head will move naturally with your spine. When you ride the wave through the whole of your spine all the way up … your head will become weightlessly buoyed above the last vertebra. You can amplify the wave again, by anchoring through the occiput at the base of the skull, which will also open the cranial structure. Sense the wave beyond your structure by presencing through the beyond.

If your knees lock, it means that you lost the anchor of the sacrum, and the lower back compressed. Use your next exhalation to anchor the sacrum again, which will release your lower back, leaving the knees extended but not locked. Likewise, there is no need to bend the knees to come up, as long as the sacrum remains adequately anchored, which will prevent you from compressing your lower back. In fact, you will feel the elongation much better if you do not allow your knees to bend. However, as always, if you are in pain you must use your own discretion as to whether to bend the knees slightly upon coming up.

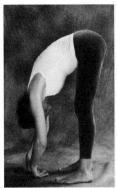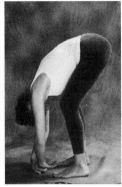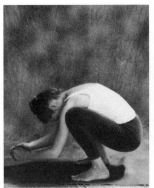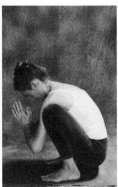

Standing pour forward ending position, followed by a squat

When the wave lifts the thoracic spine, it feels like the curvature almost inverts, so that you feel the spine rising up through your back, not behind you. Your shoulder blades will fall gently downward as the spine extends. The arms will continue to float, in pendulum-like spirals, on the way up. When the arms drink in the energy released from the spine, the heart center opens, expressing this energy into the world. In this way, the arms serve to anchor the portal of the heart open.

Variation: With squat

You can add a squat at the bottom of the pour forward when your head is down and the buttocks up. You may need to widen your stance in order to bring your torso and arms between the legs. The first few times, you may want to hold onto a pole or stationary object that can support your weight, until you learn to open and balance in this position. For fun, you can also try this counter-balancing with a partner. However, if your pelvis should fall backward from the squat, your mat will not be more than a couple of inches away, so no need to worry.

It is crucial to keep the heels down while bending the knees, inverting the spine so that the head comes up as the buttocks lower almost to the ground. The arms can come into prayer position, palms together. The anchoring of the sacrum is facilitated by this position. As you elongate your spine, the upper torso balances your structure so you don't fall backward. The squat also serves as a wonderful practice for pregnant women in preparation for birthing.

After enjoying several elongations in this position, come back to the pour forward position (head down, buttocks up) on your next exhalation by pressing down through the heels. Extending your legs should feel smooth and effortless.

From this position, do a few more elongations, moving toward the balls of your feet on the inhalation and extending the back of the knees as you exhale. Continue pouring up to standing as described above, anchoring through the sacrum.

If you feel any strain in your knees when coming down into the squat, reverse the movement and come back to standing. You can try again several days later after doing the pose without the squat, which will continue to open your joints and prepare you for the full realization of the pose.

Finish with a few quick spinal releases.

Follow-up gravity-reference scan

What did you notice as a result of this practice?

- Do you will feel more openness in your structure?
- Do you feel planted in the ground from the waist down? And lighter from the waist up?
- Do you feel less density in your upper back?
- Are your shoulders resting comfortably back and down?
- Does your head float over your spine?
- Do you feel more freedom in your pelvis or a sense of floating over your legs?
- Is your neck more relaxed?
- Do you feel more energy flowing through your arms and hands?
- Does it seem like the belly flattened without holding it in?

Questions to reflect on to deepen the inquiry:

- Have you noticed how tensing toward an accomplishment like going forward inhibits your movement?

- When you sense this, does the efforting stop?
- When you give up the efforting, can you find your own deep yearning?
- How does it feel when the "yearning" does the work for you?
- How does it feel when you open to receive space and light throughout your structure?
- As you open, does your presence extend beyond your structure, into the "whole" of space?
- Does extending your presence—kissing back—enhance your enjoyment?

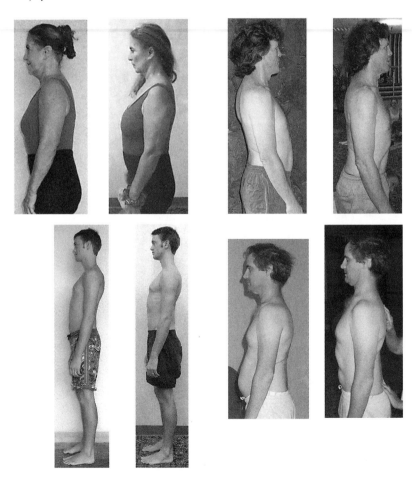

Before and after photos from a Somatic Learning workshop. Notice especially the opening space between the neck and shoulder.

Reka's Story: Beyond Apparent Limitation

In my life, I've never before experienced a discipline to which I'm drawn purely out of a love for the freedom that I receive from it. It allows me to come to a time and space that's just for me; I can't think of any other way in which I meet myself so fully. Even though I do other things in a solitary way, like jogging or swimming, I am never as completely connected as when I'm practicing Somatic Learning.

I remember how long it took to establish my own personal practice when I first started. Many challenges came up in terms of creating time and a practice space within my relationship with my partner. At times I even wonder how it is that I ever created a practice for myself. I'm not the kind of person who is diligent enough to come to something every day with such dedication. The practice just pulls you along, and if you follow, it continues to open: it's not something you have to negotiate.

What makes Somatic Learning thoroughly unique is that it brings a sense of embodied richness to how the breath moves throughout everything and connects me to all that is. This is such a contrast to how I felt coming into my practice. Even though there are times that I still regress, when I come back to my practice I wonder, "How could I have forgotten how rich it can be?" Just to function using only half of my lung capacity feels like I am cheating myself: and the practice is that reminder.

Through my practice, I found a new way of responding to challenges and crises. For one thing, I can sense the meaning of everything in the context of the whole of my life. Before I really developed the Somatic Learning practice I fixated on what's not working—what's failing. Now there's a sense that things are flowing and functioning beautifully.

For example, even as I sit here and speak I notice where it is I'm contracting myself around the need to talk into the recorder. Somehow I am creating tension through my system, and I can recognize how that feels, and I respond with sensing and breathing as I do during the practice: just letting the breath move through me.

I can also recognize when I abandon myself. The lapses of attention can sometimes be for ten minutes before I recognize them, and the realization of self-abandonment comes over me. This is such a gift, even if it takes me a while to realize it. It's a gift to be able to have this self-referencing capacity, and I notice when I'm not fully present in the here and now.

To give an example of something I have been working on: my right foot has a congenital deformity. My weight tends to fall on the arch, and it collapses. Without bringing awareness to how I can feel gravity through the foot, that gravity becomes burdensome, and my weight compresses and congests my whole right side. When I sense the gravity moving through me, everything opens up.

But this isn't about fixing my foot. The foot is part of the whole of movement. With omnidirectional awareness, I sense movements within movements throughout my entire system. When I sense the lines of force that interpenetrate through the earth and myself, the structure of my foot no longer constrains me. A wall seems to disappear when I open to this level of differentiation: it's almost like I can go right through the wall. The whole pattern of pain that I have felt through my right side, through my pelvis, abdomen, right breast, shoulders, and even my cranium, dissolves. A sense of spaciousness occurs everywhere simultaneously.

Her whole body shape-shifting, without thought or hesitation.
The upright, muscled water that she is
Molded by the rocks beneath her feet,
recapitulates the history they contain of life on this planet,
the primordial ebb and flow of its undulating pulse,
the briefest out-breath of human touch upon it,
in a gushing forth of vertical time.
    —*Risa Kaparo, from the poem-song "Water"*[1]

CHAPTER 10

Anytime Anywhere Practices: Walking

The description in the epigraph above of my daughter walking barefoot on the ancient rock surfaces of the Grand Canyon depicts the way that we can move through the world presencing spaciousness in full communion with nature. I moved to Kaua'i to raise her where she could grow up safely, bare to the elements, to nourish her in a self-sustaining communion with the natural world through her developmental years. For those of us who grew up like me in an urban environment, it is possible to live into the same kind of freedom, aliveness, and communion with all of nature, through the processes of differentiation and presencing. The Somatic Meditations provide a way of learning through "the body" by engaging somatic intelligence. Somatic intelligence involves all forms of perception in a "here-now, at-no-distance" mode of functioning.

The sacrum anchors the portal that aligns us with an infinite source of energy and renders ever-greater freedom and aliveness. From this alignment we can sense our interconnectedness not just with the Earth, but with the movement of all the heavenly bodies and the vastness of space. Likewise, proprioception serves as an anchor in somatic intelligence, aligning all modes of perception (visual, acoustic, olfactory, gustatory, and tactile), as well as meaning-making (feeling, thinking, anticipating, and remembering) to function in the immediacy of the present. In fact, it is what enables us to extend our presence dimensionally, to fully embody consciousness in an awakened state, here and now.

Without that anchor, thought cannot overcome the incoherencies embedded in its own structure. And visual perception often functions incoherently by trying to replace our proprioception. Just like a lens can polarize light, rendering it more coherent and assimilable to our eyes, proprioception can polarize all modes of perception, so they function more coherently and render the whole field of meaning more intelligible to us. Through proprioception, somatic intelligence sustains its groundedness in the present.

As these practices have already demonstrated, "the body" does not have to be a distraction in meditation; it can actually serve as the ultimate learning environment for meditation because it provides the subtlest feedback ever imagined. After all, you would not learn to swim on dry land or walk on the moon. You need water and gravity to provide real-time feedback to hone these processes. Likewise, in receiving the gift of our birthright, the body we were born into, we have the most favorable conditions to open the mind.

So far, these meditations have primarily explored the realm of "intrinsic movement." This chapter is devoted to presencing in the realm of "movement through space," utilizing the differentiated awareness we developed through exploring intrinsic movement.

I recently participated in a meditation retreat and was surprised to see, after a week, people still "watching themselves walk" during walking meditation periods. They were trying to either control it, slow it down, or find balance, looking for the ground "down there somewhere," watching an image of themselves in their mind's eye.

Having taught walking meditation for decades, I know that given even a few minutes of instruction each day in the meditation of walking, participants could have an exponential change in their meditation over seven days. They do not need to wait decades or years to attain this level of awareness. Each day they can make further differentiations to extend their presence.

One of the inherent problems with "focusing"—or replacing proprioception with the arguably more developed visual mode of perception—is that as soon as you need to turn your focus to some other activity you lose awareness. Proprioception does not require focal awareness, since it doesn't create an observer to focus on something inwardly or outwardly. Since proprioception can integrate with multiple modes of intelligence, it does not hamper your ability to focus attention elsewhere. In fact, it enhances your ability as it grounds and extends your presence into ever-greater depths of your silent experiencing, allowing you to live into the inquiry.

When I am teaching, I like to extend the practice of walking meditation to include dialogue, in order to demonstrate and discover the freedom of "mindfulness" in the Somatic Meditations.

While dialoguing with someone as I extend presence in a walking meditation, subtler and subtler realms of meaning open to me. If I am too "focused" on what the other is saying, my trajectory as I am orbiting "meaning space" may become skewed toward the verbal levels of thought (the higher orders of abstraction). When I get caught up in the gravitational pull of these trajectories of thought, I fall back into a mode of "doing"—which may translate into getting lost in "the past," in "stories," or talking too much.

When the silent level of experience lights up from within, our somatic intelligence becomes sustainably self-sensing, self-organizing, and self-renewing. Being awake on the silent level of experience allows new insights to reveal themselves on the clear surface of awareness. These insights are not automatically subsumed into concretizing "channels" of thought, since the whole playing field of meaning is continuously re-leveled.

Let striving give way to the opening … like taking off cumbersome clothes so you can swim more freely. This "discipline" is not an act of will. The layers shed themselves. It is the yearning for the beyond—the emptiness—that does all the work. I grow like a plant toward the light. The skin—whatever I am holding onto—sheds, simply because it no longer fits. It falls away effortlessly. Each new layer takes me deeper into the emptiness or, paradoxically, into the undifferentiated wholeness, the implicate order, as Bohm would say. This process is what I refer to as proprioceptive illumination.

Slow-Motion Walking

In this meditation we slow down the walking for the purpose of differentiating, as if you had many more frames per second of awareness.

Instructions

Start with a short gravity-reference scan (standing). Sense the ground supporting you. Note any differences in the way your right and left sides receive the support of the ground. Notice any holding. Notice what moves as you breathe.

When you feel ready, play with shifting your weight—not as an object from one leg to another, but as if you were pouring the liquid crystalline matrix of your bones down like salt crystals through an hourglass, first through one leg and then another.

Coming into walking position: While continuing to sustain your presence and rootedness into the ground from the leg you just poured through, allow the now-"empty" leg to swing forward from the sacrum, weightlessly. It will fall within one foot's length in front of the other foot, around hip distance apart.

See what happens when you come in contact with the ground. Let your leg connect to the ground, and then feel the support of the ground flowing all the way through you. Try not to impose your idea of walking upon your movement, which would locomote you like an object through space.

Note that if you enter into a visually dominant perceptual mode, the ground appears far away, "down there somewhere." If you sense proprioceptively, the contact with the ground can be felt everywhere at once. Gravity pulls you toward the center of the Earth, and since the ground breaks your fall, an opposing force rises up through your structure. Sense the ground supporting you through your entire skeleton. Entrust your support to the ground so that you don't have to hold yourself anywhere.

Experiment with closing your eyes. This not only reduces the distraction from visual perception but also helps to engage proprioceptive awareness. As you make contact with the ground, if your leg lands empty, how does it fill with support as your weight comes into that leg? Gradually let your eyes open, but without focusing. Just receive, so that you don't use your eyes like pincers grasping at things. Let the world come to you, through you, while you extend your presence to meet it, sensing through your tissue. Play with seeing without objectifying yourself by identifying with images.

With your eyes open, find your way back to a place to sit again. Take a few moments to reflect on your experience without going into a mechanical mode of thinking. Take a moment to reflect on your practice in writing, allowing the silent level of your experience to flower into words, so that you give expression to what arises from the depths of your somatic intelligence.

Walking with Arm Wheel

Instructions

We begin the walking meditation using the arms to vivify the movement through the spine and legs.

Start from standing in neutral position. Begin with a quick spinal release from standing (with small knee bend). This time as the sacrum anchors, allow the lower arms to float upward without lifting the shoulders so that the forearms float hip distance apart, parallel to the ground, palms facing upward. The movement is not initiated through the arms, but occurs as a consequence of the center lowering.

Use your arms to vivify how you draw the horizon through your center, as the energy comes through your structure and pours out your back. The arms mirror this "wheel-like" movement, sliding along the sides of your waist and down the sacrum as it anchors. This anchoring allows you to receive support up through the forward leg, filling it and rendering the rear leg weightless. Once the rear leg is weightless, it is free to swing forward as an extension of the downward release of the sacrum. This movement is not initiated through the legs, but from the base of the spine.

As the arms circle up toward the horizon, the empty leg swings forward from the momentum of the movement—and naturally falls heel to toe within the length of the foot. The foot lands empty. It will not naturally fall further forward, unless you lift the leg muscularly. Let the new front leg fill from the ground up, as you receive the support of the earth. Savor your connection with the ground through your back leg as long as

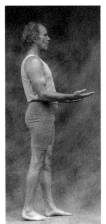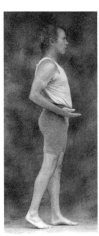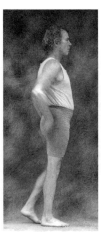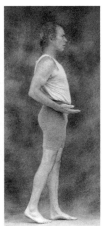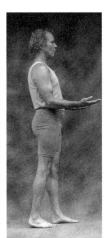

Using the arms to help draw the horizon through one's center

you can. The ground comes to you—you are not going to it. If you feel the earth hurled at your feet, you will never lift your weight from the ground.

> The world will freely offer itself to you to be unmasked. It has no choice; it will roll in ecstasy at your feet.
> —*Franz Kafka, from "Senses"*[2]

Do not initiate this walk from your legs, but from your center. The legs move like spokes of a wheel emanating from the center. Unlike a biped, plodding from leg to leg, the walk flows as though you were one wheel spinning in continuous connection with the ground.

Note: The knees should be relaxed but not bent. If you bend the knees you may wind up pushing off the ground with each step, loading the knee with weight. Remember that the knee functions best as a weight-transfer joint … not a weight-bearing joint. Loading the knee with weight as you walk is dangerous (like an accident waiting to happen) and can lead to long-term degeneration in the joint. If the weight goes into the knee joint it means that you have lost the anchor of the sacrum. Likewise, if your knees lock, you have lost the anchor of the sacrum. Remember there is a reciprocal relationship between the knee and the sacrum: if you lose one, check the other (i.e., if your lower back is tight, your knees will be either locked or weighted).

Finish with a gravity-reference scan.

Implications

This represents a major inversion from the common experience of walking. Most walking is degenerative, because the weight falls forward into each step. When you hit ground, your structure absorbs the impact, causing compression in the joints from heel to head. Alternatively, when the leg lands empty with each step, decompression occurs in the joints as the spine elongates, lengthening the soft tissues. Your perception changes also. Instead of you moving through space, it feels like space moves through you, just like the horizon.

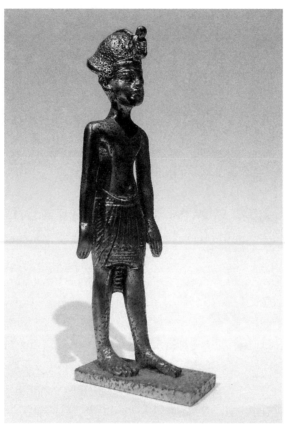

Statue depicting the stance of an
ancient Egyptian. Figure by A. Arthur Altman.

Let the wheel of the arms continue to mirror the wheel of the legs, helping to draw space through you. Drop the sacrum and release the leg forward. After some practice with the arm wheel, you can release the arms and continue the walking meditation, allowing the arms to hang from your shoulders like two pendulums. As long as the spine stays extended, there will always be space under the armpits. Vanda referred to this openness as space for a salt bowl, the kind that you find on most Italian tables. Just like with the leg, the natural swing of the arms is not initiated from the arms but results from the release of energy through the spine and the momentum of the movement in the freely hanging arms.

If the leg lands empty, you are much less prone to sprain, twist, or compression injury. You are also less likely to fall, as you are not "coming down" from above. This is why balance improves. In the martial arts, the leg always lands empty to ascertain whether the ground will actually support you before giving it your weight and possibly falling into an ambush. This caution also prevents losing one's balance on uneven terrain. When you can receive all the support from the ground through one leg, the unweighted leg is left free for other maneuvers.

The ancient Egyptians believed themselves to be the sacred space where the heavens and earth meet—an embodiment of a living god walking on this Earth. You can see this reflected in their art.

Natural Walking

Instructions

This practice carries the awareness from the slow-motion walking meditation into a more natural pacing.

To increase the speed of the walking, do not return to using more effort; this will only bring you back into old tensional patterns. Simply

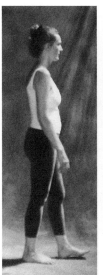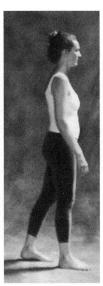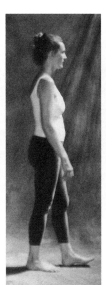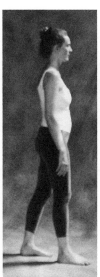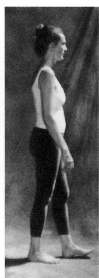

let the wheel spin faster as the earth continues to come to you. Let space enfold through you, so you do not have to move. Let the horizon continue to come through your eyes, as it pours through your navel and out the other side....

Walking Uphill

This practice demonstrates another inversion from what people normally experience when walking uphill. Here it is most obvious from where the step initiates and whether the leg swings or is lifted. If you lean forward into the steepness, lifting the leg, you have to push down on it to pull yourself up. Let go of the idea that you need to pull yourself up, as that will be like paddling upstream. Instead, lean back a bit, keeping the weight supported through the back leg. Relax the efforting. If you let the ground come to you, it will meet you more than halfway.

Walking Downhill

This represents a dangerous opportunity. If you do not adjust to the incline of the landscape, you will fall with each step ... exacerbating any pain and inflammation in the joints. To adjust for the descent, use the spinal release, bending your knees slightly so that you sit back.

Imagine that your legs are the blades of an old-fashioned water wheel. The surface of the water is just below the level of your feet. As you step, the blade turns and fills with water that then begins to empty as the wheel continues behind you, becoming light again as it rises above your waist and head. Continue to extend your presence through each leg, turning the wheel through the dense water. This extension of presence will support your steps so you don't feel like the earth is falling out from under your feet as you barrel downhill.

Going up and down steps is similar to going uphill and downhill. Play with it until you can sense the ground supporting you through the standing leg. Start slowly at first, especially if you have problems in the joints of the leg and hip.

Ideokinetic Movement

Ideokinetic movement refers to physical movement not induced by the stimulation of muscles but by the imagination. Do not intentionally engage your muscles to accomplish a task. Let the image have its way with you. Your somatic intelligence is capable of self-organizing. It makes many subtle changes that you cannot do by direct muscular initiation.

A good example of the method of Ideokinesis[3] would be imagining a skull cap filled with pet ants who are dragging the cap as they crawl up the back of your skull to the top of your head. Can you sense movement in your head without having initiated it muscularly? How does your skull feel? In a similar way, let your imagination play with the following Walking Somatic Meditations.

Large wheel

Imagine you are walking inside a large wooden wagon wheel. The legs swing from the axle at the center of the wheel. As you receive the support of the ground, it pulls the wheel toward you so that the place where your leg landed forward now comes back under you.

Becoming a walking skeleton

Imagine yourself as a skeleton walking without muscles. Enjoy what this idea does to your walking.

Sensing the pelvis as a bowl

Imagine your pelvis to be an actual bowl full of water. Play with walking that does not spill the water.

Running

It is obviously beyond the scope of this book to teach running; however, for those already engaged in the activity of running, I would

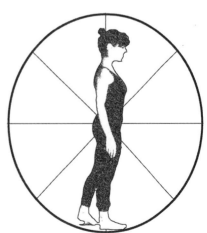

like to offer a taste of how to extend the somatic awareness practices in the book to a running practice. It often feels painful to watch runners at the side of the road do such violence to themselves in the name of fitness. I feel such compassion for the poor souls who show up in my practice to avoid knee and hip replacements, having invested so much energy in doing what they thought would keep them fit.

If you are running now, come into the run by letting the wheel spin faster (see above), not by making more effort. Feel the rebound rising like a wave through your spine, head, arms, and beyond as you extend through your back leg. If you feel compression in your joints, you are landing too weighted. Stop before you do more damage to your joints. Slow the movement down to a walk again until you can receive the ground hurled at your feet. Distinguish the difference between this effortless stride and how it feels when you are "pounding the pavement"—basically "falling forward" with each step.

Be especially mindful to release into the rebounding wave any tension you hold in your upper torso. Catch the updraft of wind under your wing tips from the medial edge of your scapulae (shoulder blades) to the lateral edge of your fingers. If you maintain the "hair's breadth" of space between your back and scapula, your arms will float weightlessly like wings on the air currents. Ride the wave of energy released from the elongation of your spine out your arms so it does not collapse back in on your spine, creating density.

Even when you are running along a "straight" path, and especially when you are running in circles around a track, do not let the subtle centrifugal and centripetal forces be lost on you. Use the dynamics of these forces as you do gravity to carry you effortlessly. Tune into the momentum of the waves of movement through your structure and the natural rhythm of your breathing without strain.

The momentum of natural running will propel you into landing first on the forefoot. What I am describing here is referred to as barefoot running or forefoot running. Most running shoes are designed to stabilize the foot while running heel first—but this creates significant compression in the joints. Several companies now make running shoes for forefoot running with full flexibility to roll through the foot, diminishing compression. However, you still need to avoid unforgiving surfaces like concrete and asphalt.[4]

Implications

In running, the amplified feedback will make even more apparent the difference between the experience of space moving through and extending you rather than you merely moving through space. Commit yourself to waking up from your "mechanistic" dream each time you find yourself "locomoting" the object body through space, and lucidly invert your participation—to awaken in "the new life."

> … and running
>
> the pavement hurled underfoot, pavement
>
> burning through our shoes
>
> and running
>
> into the center of the flame
>
> There, sheltered by the fire
>
> we stop
>
> see into the eyes of the other
>
> find ourselves
>
> in the new life
>
> The sun rises in the evening.…
>
> —*Risa Kaparo, from the poem "Overtones"*[5]

Through the Walking practices we discover how the spine elongates in relationship to the ground as we move through space. We can sense the ground's support coming up through our entire structure if the breathing is not constrained by habitual tensions. By bringing our attention to it, without making any major muscular effort, our sensing alone allows the movement to extend itself. As this happens, your organs feel weightless. In fact, your whole structure can feel taken up and equally dispersed, as if, in the words of poet Adrienne Rich, your "true home were the undimensional solitudes, the rift in the Great Nebula."[6]

You no longer need to feel limited by anything in your structure. That is the play of this: to extend your presence beyond the usual constraints of an image/object-level body experience, to a process-level somatic awareness in which you can sense yourself moving through the ground, and the ground moving through you.

To see the implications of this in other activities, let's consider touch for a moment. From image/object-level experience, we might relate to somebody as a pleasant object, one we desire to be close to, or something you are going to manipulate kindly, something you are acting upon—to heal, for instance. But from a process-level awareness, you can extend your touch so that it moves deeply and pervasively through both of you, just as it does with each step you take when connecting with the ground. There is no one "out there" to change. There is only the drinking in and kissing back of the infinite through energy and form.

Also, in listening or speaking, a process-level awareness functions much differently than an object-level knowing of ourselves. So you can see this exercise as a state-shifting experiment to shift your state of consciousness, as well as how the organism functions.

British astrophysicist and philosopher of science Sir Arthur Eddington talked about how physicists and mathematicians worked to develop a description of the atom. They made mental models from which they carefully erased details that were not accurate. In the end, they did not have enough remaining to construct an image, but they did have a more differentiated knowledge of what occurs at the atomic level. This is reminiscent of the *"neti neti"* of Sakyamuni Buddha's *Lotus Sutra,* where he describes the true nature of reality as neither this nor that.

Similarly, as you erase all the ways you are accustomed to knowing yourself inferentially—such as the sense of "I'm here, you're there," and all of the images, stories, sensations, tensions to which we have grown familiar—there is a kind of free-flow unfolding. It is personal, but not in the sense of "about me." It is personal in the sense that it is most deeply felt, immediate. For instance, you feel the support of ground throughout yourself even though what is occurring may have little correlation with any images you have held about yourself and your relationship to the environment.

Walking meditations are a mode of aesthetic experiencing without purpose. They arise from the intention to extend presence in the practice of walking. I encourage you to sense the difference between walking meditation and walking with purpose (with anywhere at all to go). On retreat, I have noticed that even the desire to pick up a sweater before the next sitting meditation as the sun lowered in the sky would subtly change the walking practice, even when the rhythm or pacing didn't vary. Something inherent in having a purpose, something to get or do or a place to go, seemed to change the silent-level aesthetic experience of walking. It imbued the walking with a sense of time and distance that were not previously present in awareness. This kind of sensing reveals how psychological time and space are organized in experience. I invite you to live into this inquiry, discovering opportunities to navigate freely through the portal of timelessness.

Penny's Story: Transformative Healing from Illness

In her late fifties, Penny, a world-renowned author and speaker, had to retire from the work that she loved because of the debilitating symptoms of her illness. She has had a great deal of experience with human potential work and was always very physically active in various practices, especially yoga and dance. Somatic Learning gave her a much more highly differentiated way of sensing her experience from the inside out, which began reversing the degenerative effects of her illness. She is once again leading seminars, writing, and seeing clients.

I have a neurological problem that affects my gait. My legs feel weak, and I had bad balance, but no one could diagnosis the problem specifically.

I found Somatic Learning to be very healing and powerful. Sometimes when I have felt too weak to walk, I have been surprised to find myself able to walk and walk beautifully. I have been surprised at how much difference my inner conscious awareness makes in terms of how I can walk.

When I started sensing proprioceptively, receiving support from the ground, I began to walk very well again. I continue to discover ways I can be in my body so that my symptoms disappear. For instance, I sometimes experience tremors. Now, when they come back, I know how to re-enter myself in a way that they disappear again.

Often I come into a practice session feeling tight and tense, yet I always leave feeling balanced. My body/mind/spirit always feels much happier when I leave than when I came in. I would recommend Somatic Learning to anyone, as anyone can benefit from practicing Somatic Learning

You needn't tense toward accomplishment.
To change your life:
Feel what your deepest love wants.
What you long for will come to you.
When you give up ambition
time is infinite.

> —*Risa Kaparo, excerpted from the poem "The Invocation"*[1]

CHAPTER 11

Anytime Anywhere Practices: Sitting

The practices in this chapter are particularly important given our sedentary lifestyles. Even children are exhibiting many structural problems from spending a lot of time sitting in a collapsed posture and in a semi-dissociated state from their body.

If you knew you could actually make a significant improvement in both your functioning and your structure with a small shift in awareness, would you settle for less? The fact that these practices can be made subtle enough that you can do them invisibly in public or seamlessly on the job, in your car or wherever you happen to be, makes them irresistible. The opportunities are endless.

Even repetitive strain patterns, migraines, and the chronic tension so epidemic in our culture can be easily prevented or reversed by practicing a few minutes and bringing a gentle awareness throughout the day.

This says nothing of what it means to enhance our enjoyment of the moment, rather than simply surviving it as we wait for a better future. A question I keep asking myself is: What is worth sacrificing the enjoyment of the moment for? Living into this question keeps bearing fruit in my life. What if we can do whatever we need to do without giving up our enjoyment by learning another way to participate?

Even when we are already doing something we really love (or especially then), how wonderful when we find something that can both enhance our enjoyment and bring our performance to a new level. This has been the case with many accomplished professionals with whom I have been privileged to work.

One world-class pianist was so excited after mastering sitting elongations to find that his hands floated over the keyboard like birds in flight. This afforded him much more nuance in his touch of the keys and extended his capacity to play for long hours without straining. Another master teacher felt liberated when the daily migraines from which she suffered for nearly a decade vanished. She had simply incorporated some small shifts in her awareness. Still another teacher stopped suffering from spondylosis, the deteriorating of her spine, just from practicing the quick spinal release a few times a day.

Chair Sitting

Props

Find a firm chair, preferably flat or with the minimum slant front to back. It is better if the chair is on legs rather than wheels. If there are wheels, lock or block them in place. The height of the seat should support your thighs at a slight angle down from your hip to your knee, or the legs should at least rest perpendicular to the ground but no lower. If the chair

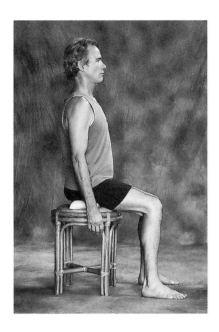

is too low or inclines to the back, simply place a firm pillow or blanket under your sit bones to adjust for it, as shown in the photo.

Position

Sit forward on the chair so that you can feel support through both sit bones with your feet parallel to one another, hip distance apart, entire foot on the ground.

Do not lean back, even if there is a backrest, or use the arm rests.

The following gravity-reference scan is similar to the one carried out from a standing position. The main difference is that you will feel the support coming from the chair through your sit bones as well as directly from the ground through your feet and legs.

If you have been practicing the standing gravity-reference scan, you can experiment with modifying it on your own, instead of following these directions. Or if you'd like, follow these directions a few times, and sense into how the practice is constructed so that you can apply the same principles to any position. This is an invitation to creatively participate.

Gravity-Reference Scan (Sitting)

The gravity-reference scan provides you with a physical reference (starting baseline) so you can more easily and accurately assess any changes that might occur with your practice.

Duration: One minute or longer

Practice suggestions

Observe "what is" in your current state without attempting to adjust your position at this time.

Instructions

Sit in a relaxed position without trying to impose an image of good posture. We want to find out what muscles are still "working" when we are at rest. There are no right or wrong answers.

Variation: Cross-Legged (Indian Style) Sitting

Position and props

All these practices can also be done sitting directly on the ground. Start with whatever leg feels more comfortable in front. However, as you do these sitting practices, continue changing which leg is in front. You can

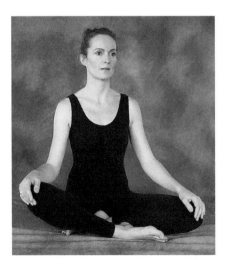

adjust for ease and comfort by using a firm support such as a block, folded blanket, or cushion under the sit bones to lift the pelvis, changing its angle to the knee. You can also prop up one or both legs as needed, if you feel a pull in your groin. However, if you still feel stress in your groin or in your hip, knees, or ankle joints, then do not practice in this position for now. Try again after doing the practice a number of times in the chair, as you will continue to become more fluid in adapting to other positions.

Questions and observations to reflect on

- Notice any areas of pain or discomfort.
- Sense your weight distribution—what percentage of your weight falls on the left versus right leg?
- How much weight is supported through your sit bones versus how much is supported through your feet?
- Do you lean more to the right or to the left side? Is one shoulder higher than the other?
- What is the angle of your head? For example, is your head leaning forward or is your chin out, in, up, or down?
- How pronounced are the curvatures of the spine? Is your upper back bent forward in an exaggerated curve (kyphosis)? Or is your lower back hyper-extended (lordosis)?
- What parts of your structure feel heavy or hard to hold up?
- What parts of your structure feel light?
- What parts of your structure feel hardly present or externally related (e.g., your arms)?
- What parts feel relatively fixed and what parts feel more flowing?
- Where do you feel direct support from the ground? In your feet, through your legs? In your pelvis (through the sit bones), lower back, upper back, neck, or head? What is supporting your head? Can you feel the support of the ground through your skeleton, or do you rely on the muscles of your neck to keep your head upright?

- Where do you sense your muscles tensing to hold yourself up? In your neck? In your upper or lower back? In your thighs, calves, ankles? Your shoulders?
- What structures move when you breathe? Your belly? Which ribs? Back or front? Do you sense any movement in your legs or arms or head?
- Observe your observing—how does your attention operate? Does your attention operate like a flashlight, shining from point to point? Is the process of paying attention changing the way you feel?
- Now make a mental picture of your posture (i.e., the alignment of your structure) and whatever you discovered, so later you can notice changes that occur.

Implications

All your observations are assets to knowing what has changed when you do the upcoming experiments.

Finding Neutral (Sitting)

Duration: One minute

Intention

To discover a way of sitting that minimizes the habitual tension and maximizes the support you can receive from the ground.

Instructions

Front-to-back axis: Rotate your pelvis slightly forward, so that the pubic bone points down to your seat. Then relax the pelvis back to center. Repeat several times to sense the movement from your sit bones through your feet and through the top of your head as a whole. Notice how the spine becomes a little more concave when the arrow-shaped sacrum points forward, and more convex when the sacrum points back. See how effortlessly and fluidly you can change your relationship to gravity. Rest with your spine extending fully upright, with your muscles relaxed.

Assessing your practice

Do you feel greater freedom and aliveness?

Does your head move with your pelvis or does it feel relatively fixed? If it feels fixed, try this: Stop watching the movement from your visual perceptual mode and try sensing proprioceptively. This should resolve the dissociating of your head from the rest of your structure. As you relax out of identification with the image world and sense yourself from the inside out, the head naturally will mirror the movement of the pelvis.

Side-to-side axis—Pouring your weight like a water balloon: Pour your weight to one side as if you were a balloon full of water, filling up one leg at a time and then back to center.

Observations

When you shifted your weight to one side, did you notice your torso compensate by leaning to the opposite side? This again represents a "compensational adjustment."

While this is already a fluid way of moving, it is possible to experience a more differentiated intrinsic movement. This produces a more subtle self-organizing as your center of gravity changes.

Side-to-side axis—Movement within movement: Without moving the "body as object" to one side, imagine that you can open a faucet in your right hip and pour the liquid crystal matrix of your bones down from your head, through your spine, and down through both the right sit bone and the right leg, into the ground.

Just as you poured the salt crystals of your bones through the hourglass of your elbows from lying supine, you can pour the salt crystals through the pelvis and leg bones. What if you allow gravity to have its way with you? Does this intimate dance with the infinite enhance your enjoyment of the moment—drinking in the support rising up through your structure as the ground breaks your fall toward the center of the Earth, and simultaneously kissing back by interpenetrating ever deeper through the ground and space? As you sense your soft tissue reorganizing itself around a new center of gravity without any muscular tension or effort, enjoy the felt-sense of your bones floating freely in a sleeve of soft tissue.

Variation—from cross-legged (Indian style) sitting

You will probably not be able to transfer as much weight through one side as when you practice in a chair.

What do you notice from the practice? If you were experiencing pain or tension in the body, notice what is released and what is changed. What moves as you breathe?

Implications

The primary difference between the two modes of transferring weight described above is that in the latter, your structure shape-shifts far more subtly, as your proprioception differentiates movements within movements. You might sense this as the spiraling descent of the liquid crystal matrix of the bones, which activates a corresponding reorganizing of the soft tissue around the skeleton (the muscle fibers lengthening, the myofascial sheaths elongating, etc., layer by layer through your structure).

In contrast, when you pour your weight like a water balloon, the weight shift is much grosser as the structure compensates for the change. In this mode, your weight is still held "above ground." When you sense yourself as movements within movements, movement is not compensatory. You change shape rather than remaining in a relatively fixed form over-compensating for the change by leaning your weight, taking on more tension to hold yourself up.

Calling through the Horizon (from Sitting Position)

Receiving through the Eyes

Duration: One minute

Intention

To feel greater freedom and aliveness by inviting more space into your structure.

Instructions

Imagine a horizon as far as you can see. Receive that horizon coming to you, through your eyes and through the back of your head. Let the horizon in front of you connect with the horizon behind you. Keep your gaze relaxed, without trying to focus your eyes on anything. The eyes act as a lens, but the seeing is occurring from the visual cortex, at the back of the head.

If you are finding this a challenge, try it with your eyes closed. Now open your eyes slowly as though you were opening the shutters on a camera and just letting in the light.

Assessing your practice

You may feel like your head is floating—like a bobble-head doll. You might even notice a change in the position of your head in relation to your spine without trying to adjust it mechanically. The use of your surface skeletal muscles to redefine or hold a posture will only complicate any problems that already exist.

Receiving through the Navel

Bring the horizon through your center—just below your navel and out the other side. Imagine an ocean in front of you and draw it through your navel, as if drinking it in through a straw.

Receiving through the Heart

Drink in the horizon from as far as you can imagine behind you as it enters through your thoracic spine (at the level of your ribs) and overflows through your heart and lungs, pouring out your chest wall and kissing back the vastness. Savor the spaciousness you presence sensing the omnidirectional convergence of inexhaustible emptiness and luminosity in embodied mindfulness.

Assessing your practice

When you bring the horizon through your center:

- Do you feel greater freedom, e.g., does your upper back feel lighter?
- Do you feel less dense?
- Do you feel more support coming from the ground through both your feet and sit bones?
- Do you feel less tension involved in sitting upright when you are not "holding" yourself up muscularly?
- Do you feel greater aliveness, more energy flow through your structure? You might even notice less slumping or a change in the curvature of your spine (less kyphosis, lordosis, or scoliosis).
- Does your head feel less heavy or forward?

Variation—from cross-legged (Indian style) sitting

Practice as in chair sitting. When you bring the horizon through you, sitting cross-legged, do you feel your spine more centered over your pelvis?

Implications

Throughout the course of your day, when you lose this soft focus and expanded peripheral vision, you can find it again by closing your eyes and bringing through the horizon. When you once again open the lids, do not grasp with your eyes; keep your focus relaxed.

Spinal Elongation (Sitting)

Duration: Two minutes

Intention

To release strain and density by presencing beyond your structure to the larger environment. You will learn to sense the wave that decompresses your spine, converting what you initially learned in a standing position to sitting. You will feel a greater ease in all your sitting activities, from typing to writing to eating, as your skeleton supports you rather than your muscles. These practices have proven very beneficial in reversing repetitive strain patterns in the eyes, arms, neck, and back.

For men, sitting is a particularly important position to increase circulation through the prostate gland. Increasing the chi flow through the second chakra and the genital organs is important for both men's and women's health and vitality, especially for infertility or pregnancy.

If you imagine your sexual organs as embers, as we age they may feel only faintly aglow. If we let each breath flow across the embers they will reignite the flames of our passion and vitality....

Practice suggestions

Begin with Finding Neutral (Sitting Position) and Calling through the Horizon practices, as well as Restoring Natural Breathing. Use instructions from standing practice (page 218), or review Chapter 6 on Somatic Learning breathing for a more complete description.

Instructions

When you bring the horizon through your center, you will likely experience your sacrum releasing downward. If you bring your awareness to surf that wave, you will extend this natural movement into what I have referred to as "anchoring." In the sitting position, this anchoring flows into the ground through four channels simultaneously. The rear right and left channels anchor down through each sit bone, continuing to flow through the front legs of your chair, while the front right and left channels move through your legs.

As in all the elongation practices, anchor your sacrum as soon as you initiate your exhalation from the pelvic floor—presencing to ride the wave through your legs, the chair, and through the ground. Remember, this is not a pelvic tilt and is not initiated through tightening the muscles of the buttocks. Let gravity anchor you to the center of the Earth, without tensing your muscles. The deeper the anchoring of your sacrum, the more vivid the wave simultaneously rises through your spine.

Continue exhaling, as if you were exhaling from your kidneys, emptying the lower lobes of your lungs from your back. As the peritoneum moves inward, your vertebrae are free to float upward, riding the wave of your exhalation. Invite space between each vertebra. As the thoracic spine becomes lighter, allow the arms to drink in the energy released from the spine, like branches drawing moisture from the ground to the leaves.

And continue sensing up through your back through the top of the rib cage and into your neck. Also sense from your armpits, from the sides of your throat, through the upper palate of the mouth, the base of the skull, and the top of your head.

Opening the crown

Repeat the elongation on your next breath—this time anchoring through your jaw and the base of your skull. Feel the energy blossom through the twenty-two bones in the skull like petals of a flower opening into the beyond.

As you ride this wave of elongation, enjoy the felt-sense of unfolding into form and simultaneously enfolding back into the formless—what the physicist David Bohm termed the implicate order of "undifferentiated wholeness."

As you come to the end of your exhalation, let it be this wholeness that breathes life back into itself through you. Let the inhalation happen in the field of your extended presence without any doing.

On the wave of each breath, sense how far you can extend presence into the beyond.

Gravity-reference scan

- Do you feel supported by your skeleton?
- Do your muscles feel free to move, or are they fixated holding your body upright?
- When you breathe, do you feel the freedom of the bones to move through your structure?
- Does your skeleton float freely in the sea of soft tissue?

Assessing your practice

Do you feel:

- Your neck elongating as the pressure of the head is released?
- Your skull expanding?
- Your jaw freely hanging?
- Your ears and eyes lighting up or coming alive—almost as if someone turned a monitor on?
- Your organs move in relation to the breath?
- Your circulation of blood and energy or chi flow increasing?

Questions to reflect on

- As you savor this merging of presence with the beyond, does it begin to feel intimate to you … like a communing with "the beloved"?
- Does your enjoyment blossom in the savoring?

Sitting Pour Forward

Duration: Three to five minutes

Intention

Just like the standing pour forward, this practice effortlessly reorganizes your whole structure through elongating your spine. Rather than just stretching the muscles, the elongation opens all the joints, activating the lengthening reflex that extends the actual muscle fibers.

Practice suggestion

Begin with Spinal Elongation (Sitting).

Instructions

Sit on a stool or forward on a firm chair (not leaning against a backrest), with legs hip distance apart, feet parallel and resting on the ground. As you inhale, relax and let your weight shift slightly forward toward the balls of the feet.

On the exhale, as you anchor the sacrum, simultaneously ride the wave from your waist down through the legs and ground, and from your waist up through your torso, head, and arms. Once the wave extends into the beyond above and below as well as all around, allow yourself to pour forward from your hips. Do not lean or fold forward with a flat back. Pour through the top of your head like a spout, but don't lead with the head; let the wave rise out of your hip. This opens the hip socket rather than compressing the joint.

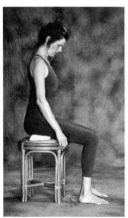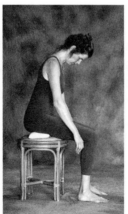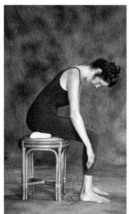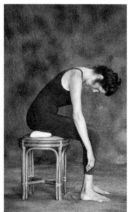

Sitting pour forward

On the inhale, relax your diaphragms and any tension you find remaining in your muscles. Suspend your structure on the wave. Let the breath come to you.

Just like in the standing pour forward, don't be ambitious about going down. In fact, it works better if you "resist" the temptation to go down, in favor of feeling the wave move up through your structure before gravity draws you down. The pouring forward happens as a consequence of this elongation of your spine and gravity, not from anything you do from the waist up.

If you are sensing in a way that is intrinsically connected through the arms, they will feel weightless and relaxed. As the upper part of the spine pours forward at the end of each elongation, the arms float, gently spiraling like two pendulums, as each wave moves through your spine. This movement originates from your spine, not from the arms. If you are not feeling them float in this way, you are likely tensing through your back and arms to reach forward, or your awareness may not be present in your arms. Either way the wave through the spine will be lost to the arms, and they will become an encumbrance.

Pouring back up to sitting

You will pour back up to sitting upright also on an exhalation, initiating the motion by anchoring your sacrum. Just like in the standing pour forward, anchoring the sacrum functions like a pulley, rooting the energy down into the ground through your legs. This draws the vertebrae up, floating them one above the other as you pour up. Do not tense the muscles of your back or neck to lift your weight. Leave your weight in the ground—where it belongs!

If you sense proprioceptively through your structure as a whole, rather than depending on visual perception to watch and control your "object body," your head will move naturally with your spine. When you ride the wave through the whole of your spine all the way up, your head will become weightlessly buoyed above the last vertebra. The upper back and neck, no longer burdened with holding the weight of the head, feel

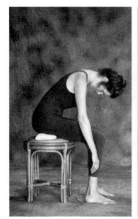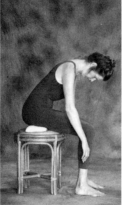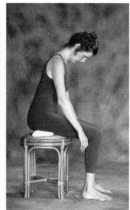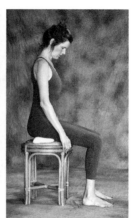

Returning from the sitting pour forward

enormous relief. Energy is freed up, and there is greater cerebral spinal fluid circulation through the spine and head.

Once again, as the wave extends the thoracic spine, it seems like the curvature almost inverts, so that you feel the spine rising up through your back, not behind you. Your shoulder blades will fall gently downward as the spine elongates. Drink in the energy released in the elongation all the way to your fingertips, sensing on the horizontal dimension—so the space in the spine doesn't collapse back in on itself. The arms will continue to float, in pendulum-like spirals, on the way up, like wings on a breeze. When the arms drink in the energy released from the spine, the heart center opens, expressing this energy into the world. In this way, the arms serve to anchor the portal of the heart open.

You can amplify the wave again, by anchoring the occiput at the base of the skull and the jaw, which will also open the cranial structure. Sense the wave beyond your structure by presencing the beyond.

Finish with a gravity-reference scan.

Assessing your practice
- Do you feel more openness in your structure?
- Do you feel planted in the ground from the waist down?
- Do you feel lighter from the waist up?

- Do you feel less density in your upper back?
- Do your shoulders rest comfortably back and down?
- Does your head float over your spine?
- Do you feel more freedom in your pelvis?
- Does your neck feel more relaxed?
- Do you feel more energy flowing through your arms and hands?

Quick Spinal Release (Sitting)

This is an extension of the spinal elongation that utilizes the rolling of the pelvis to vivify the omnidirectional wave going through the spine. A subtle form of this practice can be incorporated into any sitting activity like driving, computing, playing a keyboard, or other instrument. We will ride the wave through the arms as well, to alleviate stress in the upper torso.

Set-up

We will sit on balls for this practice. However, you can enjoy these practices from any upright sitting position, adjusting the instructions accordingly.

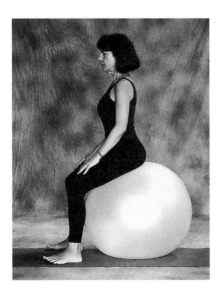

A ball is a versatile prop for sitting practices.

It's beyond the scope of this book to offer a full range of the possibilities for practice that the balls provide, especially with partner facilitation. However, I think it will prove very valuable to introduce the ball work as a variation for the sitting practices. You may enjoy it so much that you sometimes utilize the ball for sitting over traditional furniture. In general, balls will support you in staying present as you sit.

Prop

Choose a large (gymnastic type) ball according to your height, so that when it is firmly inflated your legs will make a slightly greater than ninety-degree incline from your pelvis to your knees. Balls usually are sold in three sizes (small, medium, and large) and can be purchased very reasonably from most variety-type shops.

It is helpful to place a non-slip yoga mat down beneath the ball to help you ground through the feet. The ball will best support you when you sit centered on the middle of it. (Most balls have rings of some kind to indicate the center, or use the plug to locate it.)

Gravity-reference scan

Begin with the gravity-reference scan and finding a neutral sitting position on the ball, as you would in the other sitting positions. I did not review the instructions here, in order to offer you the opportunity to invent/discover your own practice through integrating your awareness now with what you have learned "by heart" up to this point from the previous chapters.

Instructions

When you explore the side-to-side axis, initiate the motion by slowly rolling the ball from center to right to center several times. Then from center to left.

Now experiment with shifting your center of gravity without moving the ball, by pouring the liquid crystal matrix of your bones through the hourglass of your hip socket and down through one leg into the ground, simultaneously receiving the support rising from the ground through your entire structure and extending your presence beyond it. Then shift your weight to the other leg in the same way, without moving the "object body" in space. Can you feel yourself shape-shifting from the inside out?

When you explore the front-to-back axis, slowly roll the ball forward and back to initiate the motion.

Now experiment with shifting your center of gravity without moving the ball, only riding the waves through your structure.

Note: If you are sitting on a stool or the ground, you can roll an imaginary ball and get the same result.

Assessing your practice

See how you react to changing your relationship to the field of gravity.

- Do you grip?
- Do you lean forward or back to compensate for the adjustment?
- Does it compromise your balance?

If any of these are so, then try slowing down the motion and/or making it smaller. When we close the door to movement in space, we open the door to more intrinsic movement, to self-organization. Slowing down will support your differentiation—so you can go down the rabbit hole into "process-level" awareness. Here you can sense yourself as movement within movements (like the liquid crystal matrix of your bones pouring) and discern how this affects the surrounding soft tissue, etc.

Bringing the horizon through your eyes and navel

As with the other sitting positions, practice bringing the horizon through your eyes. Open the shutters of your eyelids, letting the light flood through the empty space of your head and soak through the back wall of your skull, as it would pour through a room in an Italian villa when you push open the shutters.

Observations

- Does your whole upper body begin to feel less dense or weighted down?
- Do you see with a soft focus?
- Has your peripheral vision extended?

Further Differentiations

Floating from Your Wing Tips

When you roll the ball back and your spine elongates, can you sense a "hair's breadth" of space come in between your two scapula bones (I like to refer to them as wing tips) and your back? Even when you roll the ball forward, this breadth of space reemerges. The opening of this "hair's breadth" of space floats the entire shoulder girdle and arms.

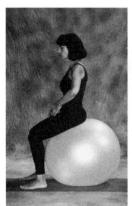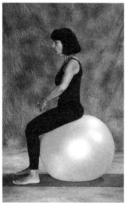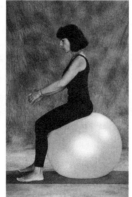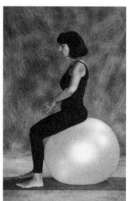

Finding space for the shoulder girdle and arms

You can extend your presence further through your arms—so they float on the waves of your breath. Start with your hands hovering a few inches in front of your center or *hara*. As you roll the actual or imaginary ball back, feel your hands drift away from your center, and as you roll the ball forward, feel your arms being drawn back like a tide coming in and out in counterbalance to your spine.

Scapula
(medial wing tips)

Implications

While the ball has proven one of the easiest places to sense this extension of presence along the horizontal dimension through your wing tips and arms, you can feel the same updraft of wind from sitting on any surface. And since this practice takes so little time—even in one breath you can extend your presence omnidirectionally—you can incorporate it into your daily activities, even the ones you perform under time limitation, to prevent the subtle contracting that happens when you feel pressurized by time.

Questions to reflect on

- Notice if your presence is no longer limited to the "object body" but extended—forward, behind, above, and below.
- Do you sense your experience all at once, from the inside out?
- Does this way of knowing create an "image/object" self?
- Does the continuum of your awareness include a more extended dimensional reality than before?

Awareness of Awareness Meditation

Begin with the breathing and elongation practices to settle the body, so you can sit with far less noise, kinesthetically. Reducing the "noise-to-signal ratio" supports the deepening of meditation. Tensing in the musculature that lives as noise in the brain and tissues mediates and distorts our ability to sense the subtler realms of meaning or "signal" and the vast emptiness beyond.

This meditation has no object; it is a meditation on awareness itself. As Padmasambhava, the great eighth-century Indian master who established Buddhism in Tibet, instructed:

> While steadily gazing into the space in front of you, without meditating on anything, steadily concentrate your consciousness, without wavering, in the space in front of you. Increase the stability of attention and then relax again. Occasionally seek out: "What is that consciousness that is concentrating?" Steadily concentrate again, and then check it out again. Do that in alternating fashion. Even if there are problems of laxity and lethargy, this will dispel them.
>
> Cast your gaze downwards, gently release your mind, and without having anything on which to meditate, gently release both your body and mind into their natural state. Having nothing on which to meditate and without modification or adulteration, rest your attention simply without wavering, in its natural state, its natural limpidity, its own character, just as it is. Remain in this state of luminosity, and reset your mind so that it is loose and free. Alternate between observing that which is concentrating inwardly and that which is releasing. If you think it is the mind, ask: "Who is it that releases the mind and concentrates the mind?" Steadily observe yourself, then release again. By so doing fine stability will arise, and you may even identify pristine awareness....
>
> If you become muddled and unmindful, you have slipped into laxity and dimness. So clear up this problem, arouse your awareness, and shift your gaze. If you become distracted and excited, it is important that you lower your gaze and release your awareness. If Samadhi arises in which

there is nothing of which you can say, "This is meditation" and "This is conceptualization," you are slipping into a stupor, so meditate with alternating concentration and release, and recognize who is meditating.[2]

Enter the vast ocean of emptiness as the beloved. And when bathed to your heart's content, what rises up and returns to the world? Does the ocean of emptiness live in awareness as you move through the world—without "drying out"?

The meditations that follow are experiments in opening yourself to this vast ocean of emptiness throughout your daily activities. Each of them can serve as a tryst for receiving the infinite as the beloved.

Integrating Your Practice into Daily Life

Eating

What an opportunity we have each day to experience the magnificence of the world as we imbibe it! A dear friend and mentor, Anam Thubten, a Tibetan Rinpoche, told a story upon returning from France about biting into his first croissant that someone had freshly baked for him there, and feeling in that moment, "I am not ready to die today."

The burst of flavor exploding on the tongue is often lost on us. In our culture, we are in such a rush to "tank up" with food. Or we are so pre-occupied with something else (social dialogue or our own thoughts, and for some people, many hours of television), that we are not very present in the eating. This is one of the reasons why food addictions and other eating disorders are so challenging to heal: Employing the power of will eventually leads to a self-perpetuating sense of shame and failure. Since the only place that change can occur is now, I must be present now for transformative learning and change to occur. I cannot be anticipating a "better future" and tensing toward it.

Eating Meditation

Though our relationship to food is often confused or perverted by cultural programming and shame scripts, as well as personal trauma, we can reclaim ourselves simply by "tasting" our experience—sensing it not just in the mouth but also as a full-bodied response. What happens if you extend your presence to "taste" all aspects of eating while:

- Feeling hungry
- Anticipating food
- Having a craving
- Satisfying a craving
- Not satisfying a craving or postponing it
- Seeing food
- Lifting it to one's mouth
- Experiencing the flavors
- Chewing
- Savoring
- Swallowing
- Feeling the emptiness in one's mouth after the swallow
- Feeling the fullness when we are no longer hungry

When we taste a fine curry, where the cook spent hours grinding the spices, preparing them in a way that preserves their unique flavors, we taste a mixture alive with nuance. In fact, what we taste is a synergy of flavors. If we taste the curry thoroughly, none of those nuances of flavor are lost on us. The texture, fragrances, tastes—ride our tongue. If we ride their waves all the way to the end, we hardly need to swallow as the food has dissolved itself into our being and its flavor extended our perception. This represents a dimensional extension of our perception of taste. It has extended both our consciousness and our physical being. And all of this happened without efforting, without time, which we create by tensing toward an accomplishment. This tasting is a process of differentiation in the here and now, without creating psychological time.

Experiment to see what happens when you begin your meal in silence. You might play with closing your eyes to deepen your "tasting" (in the broader sense described above). Then experiment with opening your eyes, without grasping. See how it feels to sit at the table with soft eyes. Can you see without losing the full-bodied experience of tasting? When you lose it, feel free to close your eyes, again and again, to help you re-extend your presence proprioceptively. After some practice with this, play with re-extending your presence without closing your eyes, simply by bringing through the horizon.

See how this shift in visual perception affects your communing with the feast of food, as well as the feast of space surrounding you, and the social feast, if you are in the company of others.

While sharing a meal with others, you can invite them to make this exploration with you. Once you have feasted in the silent-level "tasting," then experiment with inviting in the "verbal level" of experience, first by giving voice to what you feel/sense in the present. See if you can do this without either interfering with your breathing (grasping for breath) or abandoning the "tasting." When you get lost, make space to reenter the silent level of your experiencing once again, by practicing detachment in relation to your story and the desire to communicate. Experiment in a similar way that you do with your eyes, exploring how to speak and listen without "tensing" or "grasping."[3]

Writing

You can do a similar practice to deepen "the dialogue with oneself" as you sit at your table or desk to write. Before you get onto what you intend to write for the day, give yourself ten to twenty-five minutes of writing meditation as a warm-up. First extend presence in the silent level of your experiencing as described above. Begin your writing practice by giving voice to the flow of your experience … whatever rises into consciousness without censorship or editing.

Unlike learning a new language where you struggle to find "what is the word for…," when you speak a language fluently you can think in words without having to grasp after them, as the words rise effortlessly in the flow of your thinking. Just so, as you write, allow your words to "rele-vate"[4] without "grasping." Notice when you begin tensing to communicate something. See what happens when you relax the tension and open yourself to allow meaning to flow effortlessly.

Rather than trying to convey an idea from your private world into public space, play with presencing a nondual mode of "listening." Let your listening find expression as though you were "kissing back"—reaching toward the beloved.[5]

Computing and Playing a Keyboard

Staring at a computer screen or even playing a piano keyboard for hours at a time tends to incline the head forward and fixate the tiny muscles of the eye, which impacts the spine, shoulders, neck, face, and head. Simply remembering to bring the horizon through from time to time will make all the difference in the world.

When you sit at the computer I suggest integrating the elongation into what I call a "save/send protocol." Since each elongation takes the space of one breath, why not make it a part of your practice each time you routinely save a document or send an email to relax and extend your enjoyment? When playing the piano, you can make a protocol of elongating each time you finish playing a song. This practice will ground you in the reality that you are always only a breath away from greater freedom and aliveness.

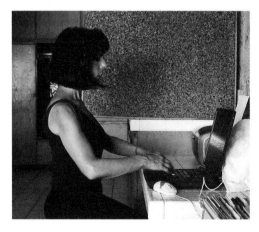

Ergonomics and alignment are "key" when working at a keyboard.

Note: Whether you are sitting at a desk or a piano, your position can interfere with how you receive support from the ground, so that you do not feel this freedom and aliveness. For this reason it will prove worthwhile to set up your workspace ergonomically. It is beyond the scope of this book to go into this in depth. For now, at least, adjust the height of your seat so that your thighs pour out of your hips on a slight decline. Likewise, the height of your keyboard should allow your forearms to flow from your elbows to your wrists on a slight decline also. The height and angle of your screen should be set to allow the reflection off the symbols to flow through your eyes and through the back of your head, in a way that allows the eyes to rest. Feel your eyes floating as if on water as you bring through the horizon. Be sure you do not have to angle the head up or down to read the screen. Basically, the same relationship of heights applies at the piano.

Keyboard Meditation

In the following meditation, I give instructions for sitting at a computer keyboard; however, you can modify them slightly to use at any keyboard (piano, etc.).

Start by following the instructions for the spinal elongation at your computer (see above) before you begin working, to extend presence on the silent level of your experience. When the monitor lights up, play with seeing what is on the screen without "grasping." Rather than focusing on the words and images, let them float into your eyes on a vast sea of emptiness as the horizon comes to you.

As you begin to process information or type, play with staying proprioceptively present to feel gravity support you, so you continue to float upright on the waves of your breath. Pay particular attention to the floating of the head. Keep checking in to see to what degree it still floats effortlessly or is held up muscularly as you type. When you find yourself "tensing," take a moment to ride another wave of elongation.

As the wave opens space in the thoracic spine, releasing the density of trapped energy, drink this freed-up energy through the arms. Feel the medial wing tips of your shoulder blades float as though they caught a slight updraft of breeze off your back. Sense this extension carry through the whole breadth of your arms like the extension of wings. In this way, the hands can float over the keyboard like a bird glides on the wind.

As you get into the flow of your work, you will undoubtedly lose this proprioceptive awareness frequently. In fact, if you set a timer to go off at random intervals (now a common feature available on many digital watches and cell phones), each time you check in you will probably find that this proprioceptive awareness is not present. I suggest playing with this from time to time.

Using the save/send protocol above to elongate the spine will break the "locked-in" focus and habituated tensional patterns of a closed system. When you function as a closed system, you rely on your own energy to "hold yourself up" in an adversarial relationship to gravity. By re-extending presence in the elongation, you keep making a fresh beginning, returning to function as a self-sensing, self-organizing, and self-renewing open system. As an open system, you transform your relationship to gravity, so it can support you in a self-sustaining way.

Assessing your practice

- What happens to your perception when you are no longer "grasping"?
- What happens to your neck and spine and the position of your head and shoulders?
- Is your mind quieter and in a more receptive state?
- Has the "signal-to-noise ratio" increased?
- In a relaxed alert state, do you find yourself more receptive to insights?

Driving

When you drive ... notice if you are "tensing toward the accomplishment" of the getting there ... or whether you are present, here, to the sitting. Does the space get smaller when you feel pressurized by time? Will tensing get you there any faster? Even if you can pass a few more cars or make an extra light or two, is it worth getting caught up in that tension? And how long does it take to release it when you get there? Compare that with how much time you may have saved.

Just by giving up the "meanwhile," do you find yourself enjoying the ride more? Do you see, feel, and sense more along the way?

Driving meditation may be just the ticket to experience a different relationship to time and space that doesn't take any time out of your day. Be smart as you experiment to stay alert to dangers on the road as you relax your tension and not your awareness. This practice should broaden your peripheral vision and frame of reference in a way that makes you a better driver.

Driving Meditation

Feel the wave, and try to ride it like a surfer so that you can create as much intrinsic space as possible in the skeleton as a whole—in the joints, between vertebrae, within the bones themselves. Then sense how the muscles realign to the changing length of the skeleton, as muscle fibers lengthen without stretching. Feel space blooming through the cavities of your head, chest, abdomen, and pelvis as you breathe. Feel the freedom of your organs floating. Allow the steering wheel's support to provide a gentle resistance, accentuating the wave through the spine and arms.

The car provides a wonderful context to learn a new way of seeing … to stop grasping with the eyes and to let "the horizon"—or in this case, the open road ahead—come to you because it will anyway as you drive. This should relieve stress in the neck as it floats your head upright.

When you also "bring the road or horizon through your navel," it may seem like you are riding a slipstream. I often feel as though I am not traveling through space but more like space is enfolding through me. Getting there is effortless when I am somatically present.

If you are traveling with another, see if you can engage in listening or speaking without losing the meditative feel of your drive. Even as you speak, you can pause to savor what is delicious to you. Invite space in … you needn't fill it up.

You may come in and out of this sense of expanded connection with time and space often, as thoughts hook you. There is no need to do anything. Each time you find yourself hooked, simply let go. This practice may turn a daily commute into a delicious reprieve.

Charles's Story: Sixty Years Young with Teenage Knees

I am Charles Davis. At sixty-one years young, I am pain-free and feel more graceful than I can ever remember.

Around fifty-one or fifty-two years old I can remember standing at the bottom of the twenty stairs that lead up to my home, in despair. I was wondering, "If I can barely get up these stairs now with my bad knees, what's my future going to be?"

I had been an athlete all my life. Part of my problem was undoubtedly the thousands of blacktop and hardwood floors I had run up and down playing my favorite game—basketball. I had begun to injure myself in grade school but wouldn't let that stop me. My dream was to play in college, but I injured myself again in high school. At age forty-five, I constantly wore knee braces to stand any length of time. Fortunately, the majority of my working life was sitting down. Another passion is photography, and I need to be on my feet. I thought about the knife but didn't know anyone who was in much better shape after surgery and certainly not pain-free.

I had been around chiropractors most of my adult life, lived with them and worked with them, so I knew quite a lot about the human body. I was a gym rat pushing weights and using the machines. I used to say that I had enough muscle to carry my weight however big I was, but if you can't walk it doesn't matter! At sixty-one, I now walk three miles a day.

Since I was thirty or so I had done intensive work to free myself from the typical male emotional suppression/repression patterns that were to my belief the source of most of my physical trauma. Here I was twenty years down the path feeling fairly successful about that, but my body was a wreck.

They say that when the pupil is ready, the teacher will appear. In my early fifties, I met my (Hawaiian for teacher), Dr. Risa Kaparo, and was introduced to Somatic Learning. Although this is not the quick fix that everyone is looking for, my condition began to get better right away. Now, after several years of training, my knees are better than when I was in high school. I always say that she gave me the teaching, care, and guidance, but I put my nose to the grindstone and applied it.

So what is Somatic Learning? I look at it this way: MDs and chiropractors are about applying someone else's knowledge from the outside. Somatic Learning is about taking your innate knowledge and applying it from the inside out. Guess what? We all have that intelligence. Somatic Learning guided me to it, made me aware of it, and showed me how to apply it in every moment and movement in my life. But it ain't over. Somatic Learning has become a way of life that I practice every conscious minute, every breath, and will until the day I die.

I call upon you, gravity. Let down
Your hair. Take me home.
    —*Risa Kaparo*[1]

CHAPTER 12

Changing Planes/Changing Paradigms

It is common for people to strain themselves while transitioning between positions. I view changing planes (e.g., from lying horizontal to sitting or standing up vertically) as one of those "dangerous opportunities" I referred to in Chapter 9. How we do it can exacerbate old injuries, or it can serve as an opportunity for developing somatic intelligence, enabling us to move in a way that prevents future injuries.

If you believe that gravity is your adversary, and that you need to lift your weight to change planes (e.g., from sitting to standing), you will tense your muscles to leverage your weight. However, you can use the challenge of changing planes to recognize your beliefs and test out new ideas.

The intention of this practice of changing planes is to challenge the old beliefs and test out new ones in the context of everyday activities that ordinarily stress us. If we utilize these ordinary activities as opportunities for practicing Somatic Learning, we will awaken a more differentiated somatic intelligence in the course of the daily tasks we need to accomplish anyway, and naturally develop mastery with the skills.

Spiral from Lying to Sitting

Before you physically begin, first practice the movement in your imagination. In this way, you can perfect the movement before you start practicing. Since most of us are already well practiced in moving our "object body" through space, there is no need to further concretize these habit patterns. Imagine yourself spiraling up to sitting following the description and

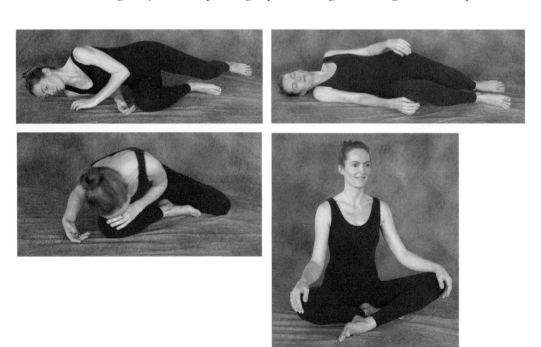

From lying to sitting in one continuous movement

pictures below. Sense yourself as a fluid medium, like a water balloon, to find the flow of this movement as a whole rather than rolling to the side and pushing up for leverage. Make the spiral one continuous movement.

Let's start with rolling toward the right. Roll your head toward your knees at the same time you roll your knees toward your head. Making a wide circle with your head, keep it low to the ground. As your head passes over your knee, continue spiraling up into an upright position, as you rotate your left knee to the left into an "Indian style" cross-legged position.

Spiral from Sitting to Lying

Going toward your right again, begin by pouring through the head and knee, sweeping the ground with your right hand as you spiral to the right, keeping your head low to the ground. After the head passes over the right knee, the spine rolls onto the ground as the legs extend.

Reverse directions: Try reversing the directions and spiraling up toward the left, lying back down toward the left again.

Variations

Donut rolls: This is the same motion done continuously, spiraling up from the ground and down again. Enjoy the play, as young children often do when they discover how to sit up naturally in this way while reaching to get their mouth around their toe.

Counter-clockwise: Now try rolling up to the right and down to the left and continue several times spiraling up and then down again. Flow fluidly and continuously through the spiral.

Clockwise: Reverse the direction of the flow, keeping the spiral fluid. As usual in your practice, notice any differences between the directions of motion. If one or both sides is/are uncomfortable, practice flowing more smoothly and effortlessly with the imagination alone. When you can flow with ease, then add the actual movement through space to the imagined movement.

Asymmetrical sitting position: If you do not rotate the left knee outward, you will go to an asymmetrical sitting position, as shown in the figure. This position is helpful for opening the hip joints, as on one side the hip is rotated forward and on the other side the hip is rotated back. As is often the case, one side will probably feel more comfortable than the other. Therefore, try it both ways.

To get to cross-legged from this asymmetrical sitting position, roll back onto the sit bone of the leg that is in front as you lift the back knee, rotating the foot into the cross-legged position and settling through the other sit bone.

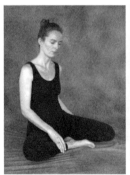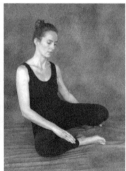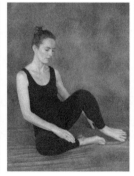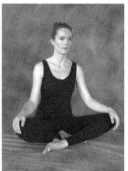

From an asymmetrical sitting position to cross-legged position

Scorpion Tail

Part 1 of this movement was introduced in Chapter 8, "Morning Practices." In this chapter you will complete the movement to utilize it for changing planes between sitting and lying. Since coming up from lying presents new challenges, remember not to muscle through it as if practicing a traditional sit-up. Rather, you will rely on your differentiated somatic awareness to sense movement within movement, as different layers of your structure move independently, reorganizing in a new relationship to gravity. If you feel stuck, go back to spiraling up rather than strain.

Part 1—Downward Roll (from sitting with legs extended in front of you)

You can begin gradually to sense the wave moving through your fluid structure by keeping the movement small at first. (See instructions in Chapter 8.)

On one exhalation you will pour the entire length of your spine onto the ground and reverse the wave to pour up. If you roll down and up on the same exhalation it is easier to practice, especially in the beginning. Surrendering to gravity, begin by releasing the pelvis slowly so the spine curls down toward the ground from the hips. Roll the spine down to the mat, one vertebra at a time, controlling the movement from the extension of your bones, especially in the space below the knees and around the sit bones. This takes the primary workload off the abdominal muscles and places it in the skeleton. Do not hold your breath at any point.

Sense how the curvature of the spine changes as the wave grows through it, noticing how the bones slide through the sleeve of soft tissue of the legs as you release down. Practice emptying your breath completely, especially from your kidneys, which engages the diaphragm of the peritoneum and activates the flow of chi, strengthening the kidneys. Use this

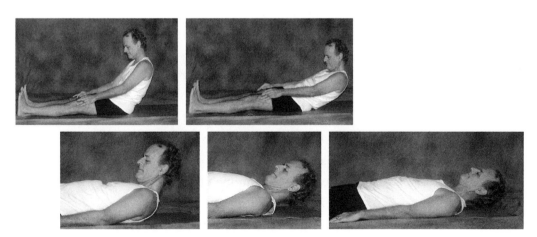

First part of the scorpion tail: downward roll

energy to empower the motion, and avoid tensing to control the movement from your surface skeletal muscles.

When the base of the thoracic spine touches the ground, keep the head curled like the tail of a scorpion and roll from the bottom ledge of the scapulae (medial wing tips, a.k.a. shoulder blades) until the shoulders come to rest on the ground. Now open the oral diaphragm by extending the space in the back of the mouth between the ears. Practice bringing the ground up through the base of the skull, rather than lowering the head to the ground. Open the space behind the eyes and at the crown, bringing the energy and support of the ground through the top of the head and beyond. If you run out of breath, pause and relax your diaphragms to receive the breath without collapsing in your structure. And then continue to roll down and elongate with the next exhalation.

Part 2—Upward Roll

Cautionary remarks: While this practice can help to decompress the spine, it also can be dangerous if done incorrectly, especially for people who have had injury or trauma to the cervical or lumbar spine. You want to avoid lifting the weight of your head on your neck, which can cause compression and exacerbate any inflammation that might be present. How do you lift the head? Initiate the movement from lower down the spine and legs, as per instructions below.

From the same exhalation, you will come back to sitting. The head and spine curl like a scorpion tail on the way up until the pelvis sits upright, where the wave turns the curvature of the thoracic spine inside out, extending the space between all the vertebrae and floating the head.

Initiate your exhalation, moving the ball of energy from the floor of the pelvis, to curl the head. Now the wave rises from the base of the spine as the three bowl-shaped diaphragms lift, all at once, with the heels, sacrum, and occiput anchoring them. The anchoring of these bones provides a polarizing force or ground from which the wave extends the spine. This allows the spine to come upright without placing undue pressure on the surface skeletal muscles.

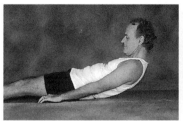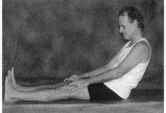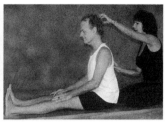

Second part of the scorpion tail: upward roll

Using the exhalation, find the diaphragm of the knee, the elbow, and the palm of the hand. Open the space in your knee joint, extending especially from the lateral side of the knee (between the tibia and fibula), allowing the heel to move even further. Moving from your bones in this way will render your head weightless so that the top of the head can curl like the scorpion, bringing your chin in. Extending the thoracic spine vertically requires an extension of the lower back. Pour the weight through the lower back and pelvis until it anchors into the ground through the sit bones when you're sitting upright.

The extension of the length of the knees renders the torso weightless. Think of coiling up, bringing the base of the sternum into the navel and spine. Extend the space between the sit bones and the knees, which uncoils the spine into an erect position. The spine and head should feel like they are floating over the pelvis, very light and extensional.

On the inhalation, remember to always relax all the diaphragms and any tension you find in the structure, sensing the skeleton floating in this sea of soft tissue.

Half Spiral and Pour Up to Standing

Begin in cross-legged sitting with the right foot in front of the left (simply reverse the instructions for the other side).

1. In one motion, simultaneously pour the head down while rotating your structure. The feet and hands will come to face the opposite direction from where you were facing while sitting. As

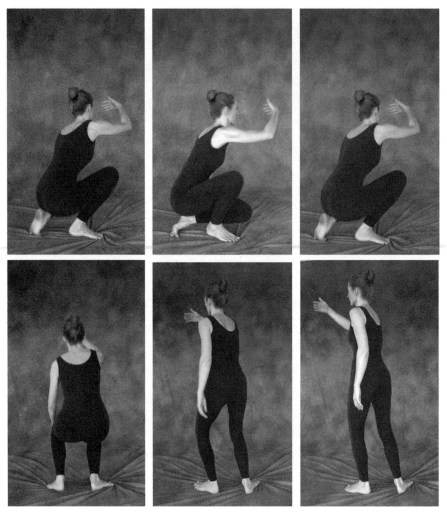

Using the arms to help draw the horizon through one's center

you come up onto the balls of your feet, place the hands down on the ground. (Both hands and feet are hip distance apart.)

2. Press down through your heels as you extend your legs; your pelvis comes up while the head stays down with the arms hanging freely at your sides. (This will straighten your knees.)

3. Anchor your sacrum and use it like a pulley, rooting the energy down into the ground through the sacrum and legs, which lifts

the vertebrae, floating them above one another as you pour up, your head buoyed above the last vertebra. (Think of pulling down on a cord of a curtain to move the curtain.)

4. If your knees lock, it means that you lost the anchor of the sacrum, and the lower back compressed. Use your next exhalation to anchor the sacrum again, which will release your lower back, leaving the knees extended but not locked.

Pouring to the Ground from Standing

1. Reverse the movement: pour down through your head while anchoring the sacrum to extend the lower back, maintaining your legs perpendicular to the ground. Keep the knees soft as you touch your hands to the ground in front of your feet.

2. All in one motion, simultaneously rotate on the balls of your feet, bringing your knees into your chest, gliding your hands along the ground, as you slowly lower your pelvis. Your hands will come off the ground as you slowly settle your pelvis into the ground, allowing your head to come up facing the opposite direction from where you started.

Alternative: Spiral to Standing

Sitting with the right leg crossed Indian-style in front of the left, place the left hand on the floor a few inches to the left of your hip, and float the palm of your right hand a few inches from your eyes. Keep turning your right hand to the left while looking at it. Your feet will turn without stepping, as your spine spirals up.

Going more implicate: Sense your bones gliding through the envelope of your soft tissue like a hand moving through a glove, so that, rather than moving mechanically like externally related moving parts, you can begin to sense yourself as movement within movements, flowing fluidly, self-organizing.

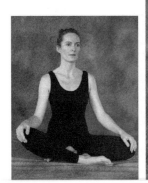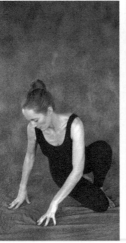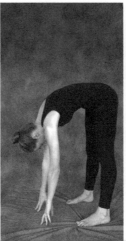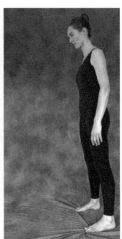

Use the exhalation to create more space between the vertebrae, by sensing the omnidirectional elongation on the wave of your breath, anchoring the sacrum and using it as a pulley so that the vertebrae float on top of each other.

Spiraling from Standing to Ground

All in one motion, simultaneously rotate on the balls of your feet, bringing your knees into your chest, slowly lowering your pelvis as you turn 180 degrees, keeping your head up as you turn.

Alternative: Lunge to Standing

The knee should not be used as a weight-bearing joint: it functions optimally as a weight-transferring joint. We use a change of direction in this way of lunging to move up from the ground, while transferring the weight through the knees rather than bearing the weight in the knees.

From the cross-legged position with the right foot in front, rotate to the left, across the ball of the right foot and onto the ball of the left foot. Use your hands for additional support as they come to position on either side of the left foot. Now reverse the rotation, spiraling to the right, as you press into the ground with your left leg, extending both legs into the spiral.

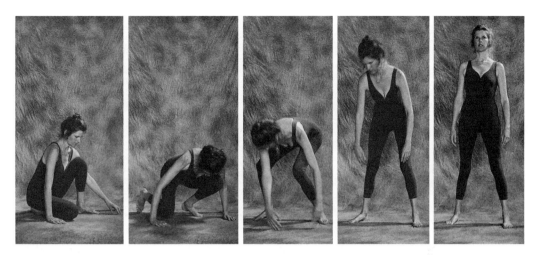

This sequence of movements avoids bearing all one's weight on the knees when standing up.

Lunge to the Ground

Simply reverse the above movement. Rotate toward the right as you squat with the majority of weight over the right foot and hands. Now turn to the left, shifting most of your weight to the left foot and hands. Once again, rotate to the right, lowering the left side of the buttocks to the ground and letting the head come above your pelvis. Bring the now weightless right leg into cross-legged position.

Sitting in a Chair from Standing

It's common for people to accomplish this by tensing their neck and shoulders, sticking out their buttocks searching for a landing, and bearing a lot of weight in the knees. In contrast, sitting can be accomplished from an elongation of your spine. Try marching in place for a few moments, in front of your chair, bringing your knees up close to your chest while lengthening your back, then sit without thinking about it. You will probably find that you naturally arrived on your seat without tensing your upper torso, sticking out your butt, or bearing weight in your knees. Now try it more slowly. Think of dropping your sacrum, elongating your spine while you bend your knees.

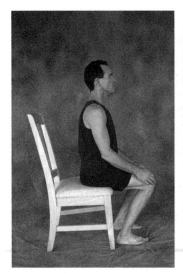 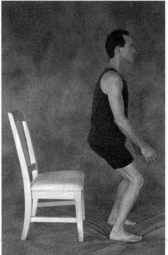 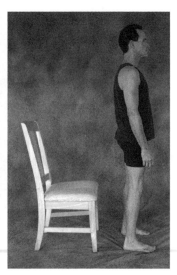

Standing from Sitting in a Chair

Instead of thinking of lifting your weight to stand, imagine that you have two valves where your legs connect to either side of the pelvis. When you open the valves the weight of your torso pours like grain through a silo, splaying out onto the ground. Your torso, having released its weight into the ground, now floats straight up. The omnidirectional extension comes from anchoring the sacrum as you extend your legs.

A quick and dirty way to activate the movement is to lift up both feet a few inches. Now gently "stomp" down quickly, pushing straight down through the feet to extend the legs. Even in this quick movement it is important to ride with the omnidirectional wave—anchoring down from the sacrum through the ground and extending up through the head.

The most common mistake is to lean forward, pulling up from the head and shoulders with the knees bearing the weight.

If you find this challenging at first, try standing from a higher surface, like a bar stool or the edge of a table. Once you can do this effortlessly, try again from a chair. Practice sitting and standing several times until it feels natural.

Implications

Partnering with gravity supports a different way of functioning within the bodymind and the world. When you sense gravity draw your weight toward the center of the Earth, you can ride the upward current arising through your structure to rise up effortlessly, receiving the support of the ground as it resists your fall.

There is a lot of talk about old paradigm/new paradigm perspectives, and these Somatic Meditations provide a way of fully embodying these evolutionary changes in human potential, gracefully and fluidly, from the inside out.

David's Story: Recovering from a Spinal Cord Injury

David came to the practice of Somatic Learning after his spinal cord injury. He started to become paralyzed on one side and was rushed into surgery, because when an orthopedic surgeon rotated his neck to give a cortisone injection, part of his spinal cord was damaged. After the surgery his mobility was still severely compromised, and he was in tremendous pain.

When David first came in he was terrified, afraid that anything he did might make it worse. Not just the pain, but fear of the paralysis returning left him feeling like he could not do anything. Besides the neck injury, he had chronic lower back pain and needed to lie down and ice his back every day for an hour or more to reduce the inflammation.

In the beginning, it was difficult to find a position in which he could work comfortably, lying, sitting, or standing. But spending a few minutes exploring each position had the effect of opening more space. He learned to relax the rigid holding of his body, which was not really protecting him. As the pain eased, he began to learn how to move without re-triggering the pain.

Besides the fear of making things worse, the fear that the limitation and pain would continue the rest of his life tormented him. David, in his forties, is the founder and CEO of a large business. As a gymnast in his youth, he had broken his neck in a fall. The fracture was not caught until it showed up on an MRI years later. Before the spinal cord injury, he was an extreme sports enthusiast. He loved skiing slopes so steep he had to drop from helicopters to access them. As a highly skilled athlete, none of his previous training prepared him for what he needed to do to heal himself. Now, starting from a place of chronic pain, everything seemed to retraumatize him. He wondered if and how he could learn to move again.

The Somatic Learning practices gave David a way of moving that was immediately healing to him. Even having begun in an almost entirely immobilized state, he found that it was possible to practice the subtle intrinsic movements that led to greater range of motion.

David often tells people that this spinal cord injury turns out to be the best thing that ever happened to him:

What I learned from practicing Somatic Learning changed my whole life in ways I could not have imagined before. I am a completely different person now. I like myself, and I like spending time alone for the first time in my life. My relationships with my kids, my partner, my friends, and my employees are vastly improved. It is so liberating to accept and love myself as I am.

I am no longer paralyzed by my fear or shame. Just as I have developed some confidence in my ability to meet myself in a way that will bring me back from pain and a way of moving that generally does not trigger it, this same awareness is leading to confidence that no matter what arises in my life, I can meet it in a way that will bring me more freedom.

What I received from Somatic Learning not only enabled my recovery, it changed how I live in my body generally. Every once in a while I would go back to thinking that I needed to train myself back into shape as an athlete, and each time I would aggravate my neck or back whenever I performed an activity the way I used to. Now I see how violent I was with myself, and how much I moved mechanically, using unnecessary force. I finally let go of this idea of "getting in shape" in favor of moving in a way that was delicious to me—and found that I do not hurt myself when I am sensing my movement in this way.

Through this self-sensing, David could see how he pressured himself, not just in movement, but also generally in life.

The biggest difference I've seen from Somatic Learning comes from what Dr. Kaparo calls "differentiation." In Somatic Learning, differentiation means paying attention to myself, and being able to sense more and more minute differences that, in reality, are huge.

Through Somatic Learning, I was able to learn to differentiate as a continuing process, like learning to walk away from conflict earlier, before getting caught in reaction. Somatic Learning has given me the tools to check myself. I learned to differentiate and identify how I was reacting, rather than to stay angry: to be an observer of my own emotions. That's the psychological part. The physical part is, for example, when I do a standing elongation. If I focus on the energy rising through my spine, paying close attention, I'll start to sense pain in places that I wasn't feeling before, and through the pain I can recognize a tension I am holding—for instance, between my shoulder blades. Then I can breathe into it and relax, just as I can with a thought or feeling. I can feel all the energy of the world coming to me. Gravity releases me, and as I open, the energy comes in and relaxes my effort. I have begun to trust my energy, as I sense it move everything into alignment.

It is not a manipulation of structure from the outside. My body reorganizes around the energy in a way that maximizes the freedom and the flow of energy through me. From Somatic Learning I am becoming present more and more of the time. And then everything is a gift. I am happier than ever. Even when I am sad, I can feel the hurt and sense there's beauty in sadness. I have come to the understanding that happiness and sadness are both valid experiences, just like birth and death. People are afraid of death. When you lose the fear, it opens up your whole world: you can stop long enough to accept whatever is.

My Somatic Learning practice makes everything a gift. Even my injured neck became a gift. When I was having trouble walking long distances, I was sad. And the sadness was curling me up like a bundle of nerves. This was only perpetuating the problem. Through differentiation, when I felt sadness I could accept it and breathe into it. That settled me. I was able to recognize that reaction in myself, and I would use my Somatic Learning practice to breathe into that tension.

Somatic Learning led me to start paying attention to what I truly was feeling, and to stop hiding under my fears and anxieties, shutting out what

I didn't want to look at. But I learned to look at the part of everything that was my responsibility: that's part of the gift of Somatic Learning. If I pay attention to me, breathing and taking the beautiful air into my lungs and moving through my whole body, I fall asleep peacefully. Differentiation enables me to catch myself when I get caught up in thought and to go back to what is really going on inside my body.

PART IV

Deepening Your Practice

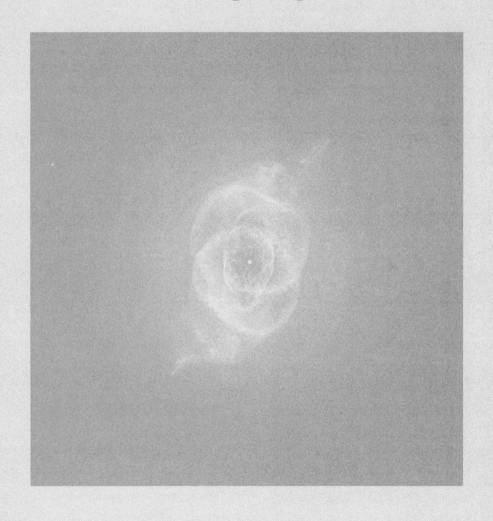

Everyone I touch is God
play us as one instrument
I have yet little experience being all I am
Reveal me to myself …

I am leaf in light nourishing the trunk
I am trunk lifting my lover weightlessly
my strength adorned by your vulnerable beauty

It matters not, which is root, trunk, branch, or leaf
only that how you love what you love
nurtures the seed of the other
that it flowers into what we yearn to become
  —Risa Kaparo, from "Everyone I Touch"[1]

CHAPTER 13

Deepening the Dialogue

Self-Facilitation through Touch

One of the most developed disciplines for facilitating Somatic Learning is the touch-work. It is beyond the scope of this book to delve into this deeply; however, it has proven so valuable that I want to explore touch as a form of self-facilitation and to at least introduce its implications for facilitating others.

Self-facilitation through touch empowers you to go more deeply than you might using only your proprioception internally. With the touch, you can provide more specific feedback to sense where and how you can release yourself.

You don't want the touch to bring awareness to the outside surface, but to awaken and release movement from the depths. To penetrate deeply with your touch, you need to receive what you are touching in a way that it no longer feels solid. To do that, you have to be formed and shaped by the movement interpenetrating you through the touching. Everything happens from the inside out. Release the idea of "doing" something "out there." As in the story of Lady Ragnell, once you disenthrall yourself from this belief, you dispel the "curse" that keeps you returning to solid form ("the old hag"). Don't accept solidness as an answer; change the way you are probing. Move into the space that you invent and discover through your exhalation. When I touch myself or another, my presence rides the waves out, opening infinitely to love. Presence the unbounded spaciousness as you drink in with your inhalation. Maximize your celebration of this moment, kissing back the divine spaciousness as beloved, with every inbreath and outbreath. For your touch to keep penetrating, to be stopped by "nothing," you must sense with increasing subtlety. Just like following the reverberations of a monastery bell, you can extend your presence endlessly. In the same way, you can follow the waves of energy and movement interpenetrating through touch as presence extends in all directions. Knowing that you can go ever deeper and "more implicate," your presence continues opening.

The touch isn't moving you, it is just offering feedback through which you can sense yourself moving more accurately. It is not the touch itself that creates space—it is your awareness and your breathing that is creating the space for you to move through. Your ability to bring space through your skeleton enables you to ride the waves more freely.

Eventually you will learn to transfer the sensation to different parts of your structure using your awareness alone, without needing the touch. Since there are places where it is impossible for you to touch yourself, you can tune into what it feels like to be touched, and learn to move from that touch, by creating an invisible partner—what I call "the invisible lover"—that provides this quality of interpenetrating touch for you. This has become the context in which I do yoga. I can move from this touch because it has become so vivid. Part of the intention I have in encouraging this self-facilitation with touch is that you can internalize the experience enough to do it purely with your imagination, and have all the accompanying sensations arise.

Once you learn how to self-facilitate with your touch, not only can you amplify your own feedback anytime for yourself … but you also learn how to touch someone else in a way that enables them to extend their presence while both participants open to greater freedom and aliveness. This avoids the problem common to many "bodyworkers" of sacrificing their own well-being in an effort to "support" another, which perpetuates constriction in both giver and receiver.

Please note that whenever your arms are not able to relax fully on the ground—especially when resting overhead, or in different positions while self-facilitating with touch—you can place a small pillow or rolled-up towel to support them so that you are not holding them up muscularly. You should feel no pulling or discomfort.

During the self-facilitation practices, experiment with using both or just one hand for the embrace. Each of these will prove valuable. While using one hand for the embrace, let the other rest on the ground—at your side or overhead. Use this arm to anchor the flow of energy. Pour the liquid crystal matrix of your bones down into the ground as if you were pouring salt crystals through an hourglass at the elbows, wrists, and hands.

Besides anchoring through the resting arm, one of the other values of embracing with one arm is that it offers the opportunity to sense the differences between your sides as you scan yourself and rest between positions. Though the whole organism will respond to each touch, the side that has the direct contact will generally open most fully. You can best differentiate new sensations and quality of movement or flow when the disparity is the greatest, as you sense from side to side. It will prove valuable to explore several functions to see how the change reflects itself in different modes of functioning—for instance, feeling what moves as you breathe on one side vs. the other. Or whether the inhale presses up against something solid on one side, while seeming to open infinitely on the other.

Integrating Other Modes of Perception

Bringing in other modes of perception will usually prove valuable. I will give you several examples, and encourage you to think of your own. You can integrate visual perception with proprioception. For instance, when you are facilitating with touch on your face, having a small mirror nearby to glance at will provide secondary feedback to help recalibrate your proprioception to the degree of change that has occurred—for instance, opening wider one eye or the whole side of your face and throat.

Likewise, you can integrate auditory perception with proprioception. While making an open-throated sound like an "Ah," you can sense any difference between how the sound reverberates through your tissues on one side compared to the other. You can also notice how loud and distinctly you can hear the sound on each side, as your hearing opens. Even following the waves rippling out from "ground zero" of your touch, with one breath, you can feel a world of difference in the capacity of the cells to resonate in a state of coherence. You can learn to sense greater freedom and aliveness through the amplified vibration all the way down through the molecular level.

Remember to switch sides, if you are using one hand, after comparing the differences between sides following a series of self-facilitations. You can also alternate sides of facilitation, which will bring balance in more immediately. This approach supports the sense of intrinsic relatedness of the arms to the movement through the structure as a whole, and helps to prevent the hands from functioning as if they were externally related to the rest of the structure.

There are particular locations where there is less need for anchoring through the arm, and where a two-handed embrace will prove far more satisfying or valuable … follow your own self-sensing in regard to this. Please take what is offered here as suggestions to enliven your own experimentation. I am not giving these instructions as a recipe to follow each time. Since Somatic Learning is a non-mechanical, non-deterministic process, there can be no set technique. Just because it functions one way once doesn't mean it will always function that way. I invite you to keep listening intrinsically and experiment. The possibilities are as limitless as your imagination.

Self-Facilitation from Lying Supine

Note: If you cannot reach any of these places I suggest without straining, don't do it. There will be other places that you will be able to hold. Take it as an opportunity to practice touching with your imagination rather than your hands.

Embracing Your Ankles

You can hold each of your ankles while bringing your bare feet up, one foot at a time, so that the lower legs approach perpendicular to the ground, but no further than you are comfortable. As your joint spaces continue to open, the knee joint opens gradually from the inside out. As you place your feet on the mat, feel the movement of your fluid structure responding to the changing position of your legs.

Take a moment to find the arches in your feet. You want to feel your heel bone extend down into the ground, opening your ankle joint. Make sure the transverse arch is open by spreading the toes apart, and elongate between the bones of the foot from the ball to the heel. When you ride the wave, you will feel more space in your ankle, and greater freedom in the

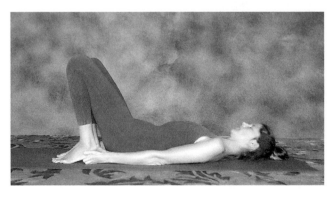

Sense points of awareness in this position.

hip and knee joints, and a relaxing of the muscles of your thighs.

Test yourself, letting go of any residue of tension you feel, especially in the ankle and the muscles of your thighs. See if you can wiggle your legs and still feel like there is support underneath you. The support of your skeleton should be what is holding up your legs, not the muscles of the thighs.

The first place to work with your hands is through your ankle and heel bone. You should be able to reach them if your legs are perpendicular to the ground. If you can't, don't worry about this position. If you can reach the lateral sides of your heels, provide some pressure so that you can feel whether or not that bone is actually moving as you elongate. The attention is to the movement of your diaphragms, and their relationship to your skeleton and the deep intrinsic movements. As you exhale, sense the wave through the pelvic floor diaphragm into the lower back and up through the thoracic inlet, all the way through the top of your head, and under your armpits. Feel your skeleton moving as a whole. When all the major diaphragms are active, all the bones will move—this is your opportunity to release any tension in the soft tissue. Sense particular points of awareness without losing the context of the whole movement.

Embracing Your Legs

Hold the center or outer sides of your knees. Can you feel the openness in the knee as the elongation moves through your leg?

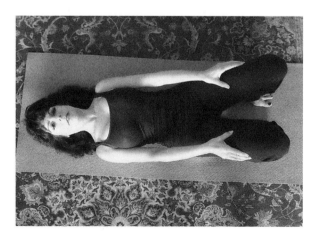

Self-Facilitation Using the Pelvic Position
with Block (or Blanket) Elongation

I give instructions to practice the following embraces from the elongation with block or blanket in pelvic position; however, you can continue to practice without changing the position—lying supine with knees up/feet standing. (For more detailed instructions see Chapter 8, "Morning Practices.")

Embracing Your Pelvis

Bring your hands to the soft spot at the sides of your hips, sensing where the head of the femur lies in your pelvis.

Give yourself some pressure to sense the wave where the leg begins. As the sacrum anchors and the pelvic diaphragm rises up, you should sense an opening right here—*vhoooom!*—as the wave moves through your legs. Sense the openness occurring at the hip with each breath.

To deepen your elongation, don't settle for just the anchoring of the sacrum. From the sacrum you can now extend your presence to the very tip of your coccyx, and ride the crest of the wave out. Lift your pelvis off the ground, while still extending the sacrum and coccyx. This will prevent you from arching your back as you lift. Even if you have inflammation in your lower back or sacroiliac, lifting from the elongation should not exacerbate it.

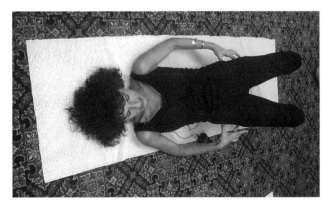

Sensing the openness at the side of the hips

Once you are up, slide the block between your pelvis and the ground. Come down one vertebra at a time from the neck down. When you reach the block, there is a fair distance more you can still go to bring the extension through your sacrum and coccyx.

Embracing Your Inner Thigh

Bring one hand to your groin and feel into the little hole at the inside where your leg comes out from your pelvis. With the other hand, press the soft tissue at the side of your pelvis. As you exhale, feel the extension of your thighbone from your hip as you ride the wave of elongation through the spine and leg. Discover how much movement there is for you to enjoy.

Do a couple of elongations with your hands in this position, feeling the movement of your pelvic floor. Sense the responsiveness through your genitals to the movement of your breath. As if blowing on warm embers, bring them aglow.

Continue to sense the movement of your legs from deep inside your pelvis. Sense the psoas, the deep intrinsic muscle that connects the lumbar region of the lower back with the inner part of your thighbone. Keep getting out of the way as you exhale, lengthening the spine and extending through your legs as your sacrum anchors. Sense the movement through the legs from higher and higher inside your pelvis to its very source. It is like feeling the flow of a river from the headwaters. The closer to the

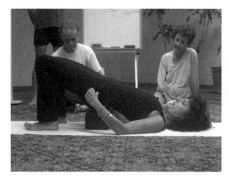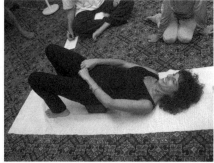

Sense the effects of elongation at the side of the pelvis as well as the groin area.

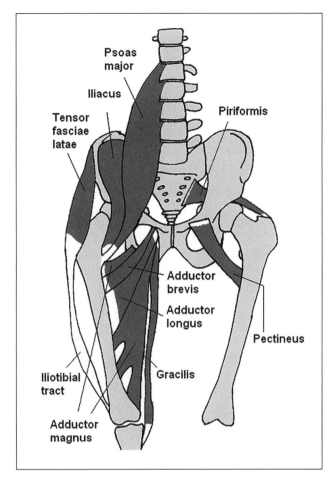

The psoas and nearby muscles

headwaters that you can sense the movement, the more the energy released from the base of the spine will root through ground. The extent of your grounding determines how far the wave extends, in terms of whether it actually makes it out through the top of your head with enough momentum and vitality before it dissipates. Sense the omnidirectional flow of force moving through your structure and beyond.

Now bring your hands back into the middle of your groin again to sense the extended elongation from there. Enjoy the rush of the wave through your spine and pelvis.

Embracing Your Ribs

Move your hands to your lower ribs. Make sure when you are working with your arms that you can feel an equal tonus ripen all around your arms as the energy travels through them. The triceps, or inner side, in particular needs attention to equalize the tonus.

The intercostal muscles create a latticework between the ribs. The elasticity of these muscles is on the diagonal. The sensation you are going for in embracing the ribs is to feel each rib free itself from the fixed structure of the rib cage. Once you feel your ribs floating down on the wave of elongation traveling up your spine, you can move your hands farther up.

The elongation is incomplete until you can feel each of your ribs. It is as if your structure enfolds back into the wholeness when the ribs move independently, rather than the outer edge of your inhalation hitting up against the "wall" of your rib cage. If everything moves with you as you breathe, there is nothing to hit against.

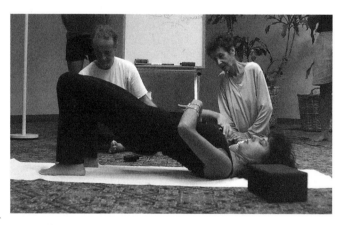

Try to free each rib and feel it floating.

Embracing Your Kidneys

Keeping both legs up, continue to move your hands up to another position, embracing your kidneys through the back of your ribs. Through this embrace sense what happens in the diaphragm of the peritoneum as you initiate your exhale engaging the pelvic floor diaphragm. Sense the emptying out of the lower lobes of your lungs from the back at the level of your kidneys.

Embracing Your Sternum

Once you have worked the lateral sides through the intercostal muscles, bring your hands slightly medial so that you can feel the area around the sternum where the ribs articulate. Create a pressure there that allows you to feel the movement of the elongation rising further up your spine. When you relax through the jaw, you can sense the wave "bloom" through your skull rather dramatically with this embrace.

Place one hand just beneath the little hole at the top of the sternum. Give yourself some pressure around the first and second ribs where they articulate to the sternum. You should be able to feel a wonderful opening in the thoracic inlet flowing out to your shoulders. If you are present in your arms, you can receive the release of energy from the spine, through the scapula; this also frees your neck and head. Enjoy the opening from the inside of your throat. This is a great time to sound on breath to vivify the change in this area vibrationally by making an open-throated sound, like an "Ah."

Flushing the Lymph and Breast Tissue

You can use one of your hands while the other arm rests on the ground overhead to get into the area underneath the armpit. This is a good way, especially for women, to decongest the breast tissue and the lymph underneath the arm. The elongation is a perfect way to flush the lymph with each breath. The movement of your skeleton in relation to your soft tissue circulates the lymph fluid. Like squeezing a sponge, it flushes the fluid out of the lymph nodes. Sense how this flushing increases the fluid circulation all through the areas where there is a strong lymph concentration, such as the groin, underneath your arm, and around the throat and thoracic inlet. You can place your hands around these areas to vivify the movement as you learn to amplify the lymph flush.

Rushing through this practice is like rushing through a wonderful meal. Savor it. Just as it is not necessary to eat all the food in one sitting, similarly you can save some of the embraces for next time. Relish the sense of leisure.

Return to Lying Supine

Once you have felt the wave move through your skull, lift your spine from your pelvis on the next elongation, and take your block or blanket out. Lower your spine onto the mat one vertebra at a time from the base of the neck thru the coccyx. Then extend your legs slowly, one at a time, opening from the hip and leading with your heel. Gently glide your heels along your mat without lifting your foot or sticking. As you exhale, surf the wave of elongation, maximizing the extension of the thigh bone out of the hip, and the bones of the lower leg out of the knee, and the heel out of the ankle as the wave extends both out your heel and up your foot. When you extend through the heel (calcaneous) bone, sense the wave move through all the bones of your foot in the same way that you sense the wave through your spine when you anchor the sacrum.

Continue to gravity-surf on the waves of your breath as you come to settle, pouring yourself more fully into the ground. In the same way that a wave flows onto the sand and is pulled back through the sand toward the center of the Earth, feel the ground absorb you. Release everything to the movement—unfolding the infinite consciousness that you are as form, and simultaneously enfolding back into the formless or undifferentiated wholeness on the primordial waves of the breath. Let breathing carry you home, grounding you to the great mother, to the center of the Earth. This practice will whet your appetite, so you won't settle for less than feeling the extension of your presence throughout your structure and into the vast beyond.

Gravity-reference scan and rest

- Feel the difference in your knees.
- Enjoy the loose opening at the hips.
- Sense your bones floating on the ground as if in water.

Remember to return yourself to the silence. Take some moments to listen for anything you are still holding—a thought, a feeling, a sensation. Don't abandon your "body" and let your mind drift off. Gradually give yourself to the ground as you would to your beloved. Slowly release what you are holding into the receiving of the ground, and let this kissing back become a form of conscious relaxation. How can you deeply embody this new relationship if you do not give yourself time to sense and integrate it?

Sometimes you may want to use your touch during the resting period, in part to integrate areas that still feel separate or externally related to the rest of your structure as a whole. Touch also can facilitate the integration and release of feelings previously held in the flesh that were loosened in the embrace. I will speak to this in more depth under the "Implications" section later in this chapter.

Embracing Your Lower Abdomen

One foot at a time, bring the feet back up to standing, receiving the wave that this initiates through the full length of the spine.

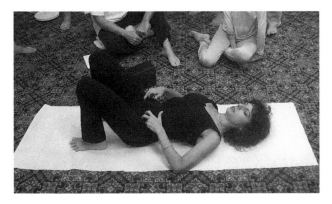

It's possible to release the fascial envelope around the intestines.

Place your hands on the lower part of the abdomen with your fingertips just above your pubis bone, and gently sense the tissues beneath your hand inviting you through them. As you extend your presence through the ground, your sacrum anchoring, the diaphragm of the pelvic floor rising, slowly move your fingers to sense your colon uncurling and unkinking as you extend the length of your lower back. Allow the organs to expand and move more freely in relation to your breathing and their own motility. Sense the subtle release of the fascial envelope around the intestines (the greater omentum). This corresponds to where Chinese medicine locates the *dantian,* or center of chi flow, in the physical body. When the fascial envelope releases, it not only allows greater movement or peristalsis in the intestines, thereby improving digestion (through the absorption of nutrients and elimination of wastes), but this release also promotes greater chi flow in all systems of the body. By supporting the organs through your touch to extend into the space that your elongated spine created, your organismic functioning integrates as a whole at a higher level of coherence.

I often remind students to "move in," so to speak, to the space and enjoy the luxury of new freedom and aliveness that increased organ motility and mobility offer. As the old adage goes, "Possession is nine-tenths of the law." If you extend your presence to take up or possess the space, you are far less likely to lose it again.

Embracing Your Umbilicus

Resting one arm on the ground overhead (or on a pillow), bring one of your hands to the navel, and press gently until you can feel a pulsing under your finger. The umbilicus always has an enormous, vital force associated with it. It was the source of your lifeblood initially and remains one of the primary vortices of your life force. Slowly draw your fingers down from your navel toward your pubic bone as you breathe. Continue sensing the pulses moving around your fingers. Keep releasing everywhere you hold tension, which the gentle pressure of your touch will help to reveal.

If you had put your hand here before you did your first gravity-reference scan, you would probably get a completely different read. For many people, just touching here is extremely painful. Now that there is so much room in the abdomen, the sense of pressure changes dramatically.

Keep releasing through the pelvis, inventing and discovering more space with each breath. The more you keep anchoring through the sacrum as you exhale, the more you disappear and allow space for all the organs of the abdomen to unfold themselves.

Return your hands to your sides again and take a moment to feel your hands and arms on the ground as part of the whole movement of breathing. Remember the danger with this self-facilitation: the arms could become an external reference to your image of yourself "minus arms." You could get used to sensing yourself this way. It is really important to keep coming back in and sensing the intrinsic relatedness of all the parts to the arms.

Embracing Your Cranium

Place one hand on your jaw and with other hand lightly pull the hair at the base of the skull (as close to the scalp as possible). When you give yourself that pressure, sense in between your ears, where your spine enters your head. As you anchor through the occiput, at the base of your skull,

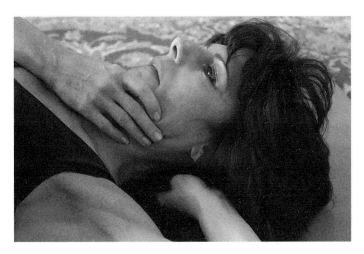

Anchoring the base of the skull to amplify the wave through the cranium

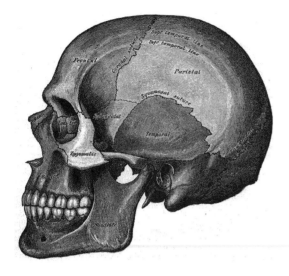

sense the movement of your elongation bloom through your cranium.

Open from the inside of your mouth as the upper palate diaphragm moves, releasing any tension from the back of the tongue and the jaw. This facilitation will most likely increase amplitude of the wave into the skull, maximizing movement through the cranium and the flow of cerebrospinal fluid through the brain, as well as structurally shifting the axis of your head to your spine. The cranium should feel like a blooming flower.

Embracing Your Crown

Press gently at the top of the skull with both hands to sense the wave coming through the crown. From this position where the two parietal bones articulate, you can enjoy the subtle movement as they open slightly, together with the release of the faux (the membrane that separates the two hemispheres of the brain). You can also relish the delicious awakening of nerve endings on your scalp, as the muscles release to the wave.

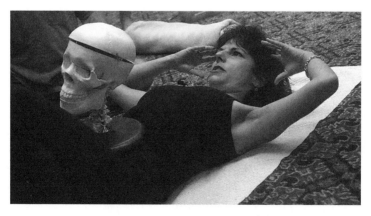

Enjoy the feeling of your skull bones releasing open like the petals of a flower.

Embracing Your Spine from Tail to Crown

Keep one hand on the crown, and bring the other hand to hold the tip of your coccyx. As you elongate, sense the wave through the base of your spine with one hand as you root through the ground from your heels, and with the other hand sense the opening between the parietal bones and the wave move beyond, through the top of your head.

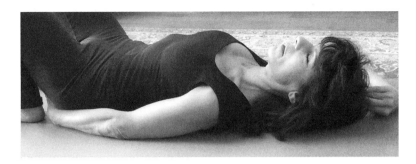

Embracing Your Arms

Once you can sense the movement as a whole, relax your touch and let your arms rest on the ground over your head. Pay attention particularly to the elongation through your arms. As you are emptying out from the pelvic floor diaphragm along the back and kidneys, continue to feel each of your ribs moving with the elongation. Find where in the wave the scapulae can relax, and open wide. This will carry the wave of energy

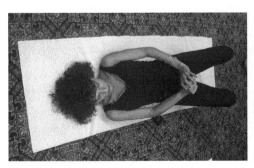
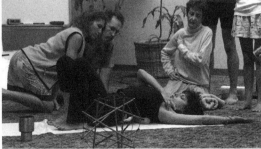

Embracing the wrist and the head of the humerus at the armpit to amplify the elongation of the arm

through your arms. Feel the energy flow from the armpit to the elbow, opening through the lower arms. Anchor that flow through your elbows, through your wrist, through your palms, and sense the energy extend through your fingertips as the wave moves out through the arms. Do not push the arms against the ground, but differentiate your sensing to feel the salt crystals of your bones being strewn like a mound of sand along a ridge, flowing down your upper and lower arms, between the major anchors of the elbow, wrist, and hand.

If you have one arm that is much tighter than the other and less able to lie on the ground, you can give yourself a little pressure between the sternum and the first few ribs with your other arm, to provide an additional anchor to extend further through your arm.

Coming to rest

For the moment, leave your arms extended in this position above your head. Extend your legs so that the pool of your lower back rests deeper in the ground. All at once, the leg extends out of the hip socket, the knee extends out of the lower leg, and the heel extends out of the foot, and all the bones of the foot respond to the wave moving through the leg.

How you return to silence has everything to do with how rich and deep a silence you return to. If you give yourself up all at once, you lose the depth of differentiation that you can bring to the silence. You want to bring yourself to the silence the way you bring your presence to the most honored guest you have received, or to the touch of someone who is greatly loved. Present yourself to the ground, don't just drop yourself off there. You are rising to meet the silence in the ground with an extension of your presence. Through kissing back, extending your presence to take up the infinite in an intimate embrace as the beloved, you can actually drink in the silence more fully. As you invite the ground and the silence through you, feel yourself immerse completely, bathing to your heart's contentment.

Your arms have been really good to you—express your gratitude by being present in them, allowing them to feel connected to the whole of what they have served. Just like you can feel your legs not just resting on the ground but also flowing out of your hips, sense your arms flowing out of your shoulders and spine, from the elbow through the wrist, and the wrist through the fingertips. Rest in that flow rather than simply setting the arms down, by sensing the wave of elongation through the arms as they are intrinsically related to the whole of your structure.

How do you know when you are ready to move? When you have re-cohered sufficiently from all the disorganizing and reorganizing that has arisen from the practice. One bit of feedback that you need to release further into a more fluid state is any pulling between or within the tissues. Continue melting until these sensations cease to exist. Let the undulating pulses and shape-shifting settle before you move. When you sense a readiness to move and feel sufficiently refreshed, relaxed, and alert, then spiral around and come on up.

As you sit, take a moment to sense sitting. Don't assume what you need to do to sit up. Close your eyes and find out proprioceptively. In other words, as you move in space don't conform to an old image of yourself to move. Find out in your moving what is needed.

> Mold clay into a vessel;
> it is the emptiness with
> that creates the usefulness of the vessel.
> … Thus, what we have may be something substantial,
> But its usefulness lies in the unoccupied, empty space.
> The substance of your body is enlivened
> by maintaining the part of you that is unoccupied.
> —*Lao Tzu*[2]

Facilitated Elongations: Quick Outline

Once you have read through the text, this brief outline can remind you of the primary hand positions to incorporate in your practice.

Use the firm embrace of your hands to vivify the wave, so you can maximize movement through your structure as you breathe and elongate.

Suggestions for the Cranial and Cervical Support

- Hold at lateral center of hip crest
- Hold at lateral, superior edge of thigh
- Hold at lateral edge of heel
- Hold edge of ribs along the sternum, moving upward until inferior, superior proximal, and lateral edges of the shoulder blades release into the ground
- Hold parietals at top of head and at temporal articulations
- Hold temporal mandibular joint once occiput has decompressed

Always return the arms to the ground, either above your head or at your sides, and sense the wave of elongation through your arms in concert with how it plays through your structure as a whole.

In the thoracic and pelvic positions

Repeat the first three hand positions above and try using one hand at a time while the other elongates. To support differentiation of the movement

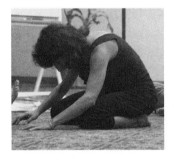
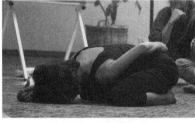
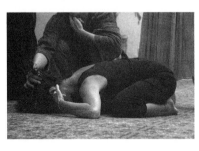
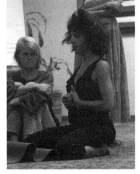

Child's pose

through the ribs, move the hands to touch both medially to laterally as well as up and down, then rest both hands overhead.

Other Possibilities

The subject of touch is so open-ended, it is not possible to wrap our arms around it here. However, because of what a significant role it has played in Somatic Learning I have hoped to leave enough breadcrumbs for anyone wanting to take this journey to find their way on this pathless path of awakening. It would get too unwieldy to describe every possibility for self-facilitation, so I have only covered the main ones to which I think you will want to return again and again from various positions. I include some photos here to give you a sense of the possibilities that abound for future exploration. I encourage you to savor the deliciousness of this embrace.

Facilitating Others

Again, all I can say here will merely reflect the tip of the iceberg of the art and practice of Somatic Learning touchwork. I strongly encourage you to seek out a practitioner of it to enjoy a first-hand experience from one who has had training.

By now it must be apparent that we practice a unique kind of touch in Somatic Learning. On one hand it is non-interventionist and non-coercive, meaning that we don't start from an "ideal" image that we try to accomplish through manipulation. Also, the touch we are describing is not directed "outwardly." As we described through the metaphor of fairytale, it is an embrace, which dispels the curse of duality. Inward and outward, private world and public space, bedchamber and court are no longer mistaken as properties of reality. They are seen as distinctions we make for a purpose. The touch is proof positive that the nature of reality has no final "objective" ground. Nature responds according to how we touch or probe it.

I know of no better way to learn to touch another with the level of differentiation and sensitivity necessary to extend presence beyond "the known" than through embracing oneself—to get out of the way, as it were, releasing and inviting the vast spaciousness through—so that we offer another an invitation they cannot refuse. When someone makes space within themselves to receive the infinite through you, you have no choice but to open and flower into what you yearn to become.

I encourage you to explore this soul-engendering embrace, not just in the context of facilitation, but also in every context that you have an opportunity to touch another being.

Rather than repeat instructions in the context of facilitating others, I include some photos to provide examples of where you might place yourself to comfortably offer the touch to another while he or she is practicing elongations.

Remember that if you are not experiencing greater freedom and aliveness in your touching, the other person will not receive those benefits either. Use the feedback you experience in the interpenetration to gauge their movement and your touch. Remember, you are not waiting for something to happen in the future, nor working with something that has already occurred in the past. You are inventing/discovering the present in your creative, compassionate, and empowered participation with what is. Start with sensing your breathing, awakening to receive the Beloved coming to you effortlessly, and "kissing back" with your touch.

Partner Facilitation from Upright Positions (Sitting and Standing)

As facilitator, you can support another in sensing the wave of elongation more vividly by sending energy down through the anchors listed above. In addition, the following placements can be used:

1. Placing one hand just below the navel and the other across from it at the back of the spine, receive the "energy" flowing through your back hand as your partner brings through the horizon.
2. Placing one hand on the base of the skull and one hand on the forehead, feel the head float when your partner brings through the horizon.

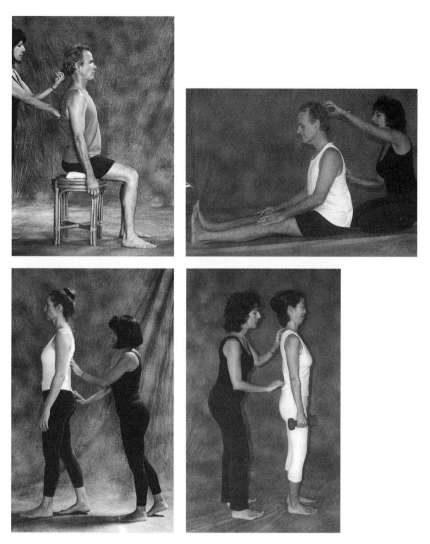

Partner facilitation allows both participants to better sense waves of elongation moving through the body.

3. Placing one hand on the sacrum and one hand on the thoracic spine, then anchoring down through the sacrum and receiving the wave up through the thoracic spine, will support your partner in creating more space between the vertebrae that lie between your hands. Do not try to facilitate this by pressing from your hands but by elongating your own spine on the

waves of your breath. As you invent and discover more space, it translates directly through your hands from your structure through theirs.

4. When you do it in this way, you make an offer your partner cannot refuse.

From lying

When someone first begins to lie on the ball, they often start by resisting the discomfort of the pressure of the ball. As you take up the invitation of the ball to ease into a deeper relaxation, a profound sense of freedom and aliveness can arise. In addition to using touch to support your partner in presencing more spaciousness through his/her structure, you can use weights to vivify the invitation of gravity to release the patterns of tension.

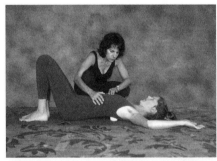
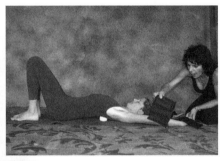
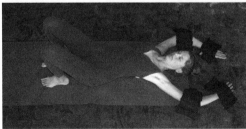

From child's pose: Partner-facilitated

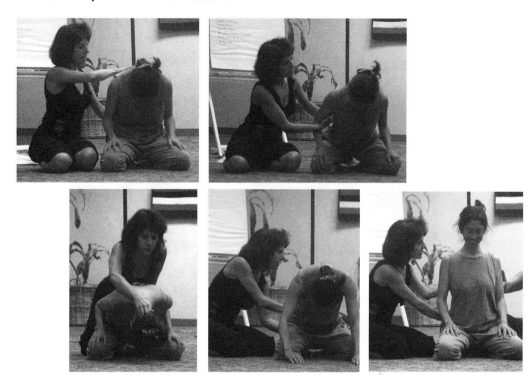

Applying touch during the execution of child's pose can help magnify the sense of space and elongation.

Healing from Trauma and Integrating Feelings through the Embrace

The embrace can be especially supportive in the moment when touch stirs painful memories or previously unintegrated depths of feeling. Since our response to trauma is often dissociation, the embrace can make you whole again by "celebrating home" the dissociated aspects of the self. As Peter Levine's somatic work has revealed,[3] when an animal comes out of the shock of trauma, in order to release the trauma held in the tissues, the organism needs to be freed from its paralyzing freeze response. This is achieved by completing the movement that had been in process at the moment it was frozen by fear. Your self-embrace can support the "traumatized animal" in you, by releasing what it is still holding onto in order to protect or defend itself. There is no statute of limitations on retrieving this lost part from its frozen state. We can meet the traumatized "little one" as the capable adult we have become, and embrace ourselves into presence. We must take up all the dissociated feelings and welcome them back home, into our "ample flesh,"[4] if we are to become whole again.

Embracing oneself flies in the face of our cultural conditioning, which only sanctions relating to ourselves as an object for a purpose, like looking good and being presentable. We have to look to the new arrivals on the planet to see another form of self-touch. We can see babies touching themselves in non self-conscious ways, naturally self-soothing, and thereby relieving stress and discomfort. But this somatic intelligence is generally lost as children become more self-conscious and acculturated. To thrive at all, most people have had to experience some form of loving touch—as it is so crucial to our survival. In fact, a recent study showed that "tactile kinesthetic stimulation" (a scientific term for touch) applied for five minutes a day helped premature babies gain an average of forty-seven percent more weight on the same formula than other babies did (making the researchers conclude that it was a cost-effective treatment).[5]

However, our access to loving touch generally becomes limited to a very narrow context: between parents and children, and between lovers. The kind of embrace that "celebrates us home" is rarely experienced in relation to ourselves. I think this accounts for so much of the codependency we find in relationships. Since we have so little experience in "holding ourselves" in a way that is self-soothing and nurturing, we are desperate to hold onto any source that can provide the comfort that we instinctively know is necessary to our survival. Learning to embrace ourselves liberates us, in part, from this dependency on another, and allows us to receive the boundless love that has always been there for us. Once we learn and accept this form of self-embrace, then we can invite another person into an intimacy that celebrates the beauty of our interdependency as humans.

When we give the entirety of this crucial element of our well-being and happiness to another, we risk spending the rest of our lives trying to control what they do with it. That this is a dangerous recipe for a relationship should be obvious. Nonetheless, it's a situation in which many of us find ourselves trapped. Blaming ourselves when such a relationship doesn't provide us with the sanctuary we need perpetuates the shame scripts that sometimes narrate our lives.

In Summation

The implications of this "embrace" go far beyond what people normally think of as "the body." We can reclaim our lives from the automated scripts of personal trauma and societal conditioning, as we learn to sustain a healthy ecology of affect that liberates us. No matter what may have happened in your developmental years, when you thoroughly embody mindfulness, the self-sensing, self-organizing, and self-renewing aspects of somatic intelligence reveal your true nature.

As we break out of our learned dependent and codependent behaviors, we can ever more freely receive love and deep nourishment directly from the infinite, and be the Love that we yearn to be, without fear or attachment. The practice of this embrace brings such immediacy and intimacy to my sense of the all-pervading, unbounded spaciousness that "Beloved" has become my favorite term for it. It is a process in which both the learned and distorted images of self—and the experience of the body as merely an object—disappear, leaving only the deliciousness of loving. Aaahh … Yes!

Dear Reader, I invite you to offer yourself fully to this embrace. Release everything. There is nothing to do, nothing to improve, nothing to achieve. Open your heart and relax deeper and deeper into the groundless ground of consciousness.

Enjoy!

To what shore would you cross, O my heart?

There is no traveller before you, there is no road:

Where is the movement, where is the rest, on that shore?

There is no water; no boat, no boatman, is there;

There is not so much as a rope to tow the boat, nor a man to draw it.

No earth, no sky, no time, no thing, is there: no shore, no ford!

There, there is neither body nor mind: and where is the place that shall
   still the thirst of the soul? You shall find naught in that emptiness.

Be strong, and enter into your own body: for there your foothold is firm.

Consider it well, O my heart! go not elsewhere.

Kabir says: "Put all imaginations away, and stand fast in that
   which you are."

   —*Kabir*[6]

Glossary

coronal

A coronal (also known as frontal) plane is a Y-X plane, perpendicular to the ground, which (in humans) separates the anterior from the posterior, the front from the back, the ventral from the dorsal.

diaphragms

People often think of a respiratory diaphragm, referring to the thoracic diaphragm, singularly. However, I refer to several other muscles, membranes, and fluid structures (that define different cavities or areas) that move as you breathe, as diaphragms.

differentiation

—Simply noticing change or movement.

—Differentiation is a core process that informs Somatic Learning. By differentiation we mean the ability to notice increasingly subtle changes or movements. The more we sense differences, the more responsive we are and more efficient our movements become. When we minimize tension, we are more sensitive.

—Learning to sense differences, movement, change. Areas that seem fixed or solid from the outside open as you sense changes and movement from within. Your somatic awareness becomes increasingly subtle as the process of differentiation develops.

distal

The point furthest from the point of attachment to the body.

embodied mindfulness

In Somatic Learning I use this term to refer to an awakened state of engaging somatic intelligence in presencing spaciousness. It can also be described as the "drinking in" and "kissing back" of the infinite as the beloved.

Our embodiment into this finely tuned feedback system (the human body) is a gift. As this perfect learning environment for the extension of presence to embody a vast spaciousness is received, our natural state is reclaimed.

interoception

Awareness of your internal state.

lateral

Lateral means "to the side," as opposed to the term *medial,* referring to "middle." The usage "mediolateral" describes relative position along the left-right axis, to avoid confusion with the terms "superficial" and "deep."

medial

center vertical line

mindfulness

—compassionate, non-judgmental, nondual, direct, and immediate awareness of the moment.

—The calm awareness of one's body functions, feelings, content of consciousness, and consciousness itself.

—Mindfulness (Pali: *sati,* Sanskrit: *smṛti*) plays a central function in Buddhist meditation, where it is seen as the critical factor in liberation and enlightenment.

Practicing mindfulness in Buddhism means to consciously perform all activities with the quality of non-attached, non-judgmental observation of experience.

nondual

The term "nondual" (meaning "not two") is used to denote affinity, or unity, in contrast to duality, separateness, or multiplicity. It refers to the idea that things appear distinct while not being separate.

organismic functioning

How the organism functions as a whole to sustain and renew itself. Our organismic functioning reflects our state of consciousness.

presencing

In Somatic Learning I use the term *presencing* to imply the embodying of spaciousness with awakened somatic intelligence. Extending presence refers to the process of living into the unknown, relaxed and curious, without efforting to grasp anything—aware of what happens in the bodymind as you ease the struggle to "wrap your mind around something." If we can be present or mindful as we live into the unknown, the infinite reveals itself to us so that we come to know it intimately.

prone

Position of the body lying face down.

proprioception

Proprioception is, literally, how we "sense ourselves." There are three main sources of input into our proprioceptive system: *Kinesthesia* is the feeling of movement derived from all skeletal and muscular structures. Kinesthesia also includes the feeling of pain, our orientation in space, the passage of time, and rhythm. *Visceral feedback* consists of the miscellaneous impressions from our internal organs. *Labyrinthine* or *vestibular feedback*—the feeling of balance as related to our position in space—is provided by the cochlea, an organ of the inner ear.

proximal

Nearer the center of the body (as opposed to "distal," meaning further out on the periphery).

relevate

A non-mechanical thought process whereby relevant meaning elevates spontaneously into consciousness following the flow of meaning. This describes the process of insight.

There is a non-mechanical mode of thinking that David Bohm referred to as *relevation*. It is an archaic English word that fell out of common usage. Etymologically, it comes from two roots: *relevant* and *elevate.* It refers to instances when meaning elevates spontaneously out of its relevance to the flow of felt significance. For example, translating our thoughts while learning a new language as an adult involves the mechanical process of looking up the word for this or that. In contrast, speaking in one's native tongue is non-mechanical—the process of relevation. An idea displays itself on the "screen of consciousness" and words rise up spontaneously to express it … we do not need to grasp after the words. Similarly, the process of insight arises from an effortless awareness of the self-arising stream of meaning. It is a process of "drinking in and kissing back"—what reveals itself to us without tensing toward an accomplishment.

sagittal

A sagittal (also known as lateral) plane is a Y-Z plane, perpendicular to the ground, which separates left from right. The mid-sagittal plane is the specific sagittal plane that is exactly in the middle of the body.

self-organization and organismic self-regulation

In the context of Somatic Learning, I use this term to refer to a person responding from his or her own natural state and needs, learning to obtain greater coherence from the feedback of his or her organism functioning as a whole in relation to its environment, in contrast to functioning in a state of fragmentation with a dependency on external regulations. It involves direct, immediate awareness of the depths of experiencing including electrochemical, neuromuscular, sensory, intuitive, affective, and cognitive modes of experience in relation to the present circumstances and conditions.

somatic

The word "somatic" comes from the Greek root *soma,* for "body." The conventional use of the word "body" in English implies an "object" observed from the outside. It is a "third-person" image of ourselves at a distance. I use the term "soma" to refer to how we sense the unfolding of life from within. I use the term "somatic" to imply a first-person, here-now, all-at-once, embodied intelligence—how we sense, feel, and know on a process level—from the inside out. This is what we are in our fullness at "no distance," in contrast to a "third-person" image of "what is" at a distance.

somatic intelligence

—I use this term to denote a here-now, all-at-once, self-sensing, self-organizing, and self-renewing system. The natural wisdom of the bodymind.

—The intelligence of the living matrix, which the Oschmans refer to as a "veritable symphony of vibratory messages."

—It involves direct, immediate awareness of the depths of experiencing, including electrochemical, neuromuscular, sensory, intuitive, affective, and cognitive modes of experience in relation to the present circumstances and conditions.

Somatic Learning

The art and practice of embodied mindfulness—a nondual methodology for awakening somatic intelligence synthesizing meditative, psychological, and somatic disciplines. Also, the development of direct, immediate awareness for how we make meaning (evaluate and respond), with particular emphasis on sensory and affective awareness.

Somatic Meditations

Embodied mindfulness practices designed to engage somatic intelligence in dimensionally extending presence to embody spaciousness. As somatic intelligence awakens, the inherent wisdom of the bodymind—which is self-sensing, self-organizing and self-renewing—becomes obvious. In this way the misidentification of taking "image/object" consciousness for the ground of reality is recognized and transformed.

supine

Lying on one's back with the face up.

tensegrity

A term coined by Buckminster Fuller as a contraction of "tensional integrity." I use this principle in Somatic Learning to refer to a structure with equalized tensional forces—one that requires minimum tension to sustain itself.

Notes

Acknowledgments

1. "What can you give that can never be taken?" Risa Kaparo, lyrics from the poem "Querencia" (song version) on the album *Awaken* (Las Vegas, Nevada: Portal Arts, 2010), www.portalarts.com.

Introduction

1. Harriet Witt-Miller, "The Soft, Warm, Wet Technology of Native Oceania," *Whole Earth Review* (Fall 1991), pp. 64–69.

> "Man's testicles might not seem like something to be used for navigation, but they were and are in native Oceania. So are stars, driftwood, clouds, seaweed, winds, birds, weather, the smell, taste, and temperature of the ocean, interference patterns on the sea's surface, and the olfactory sense of an on-board pig.
>
> "How? Our search for the answer begins in our 50th state.
>
> "Hawaii is the most isolated archipelago on Earth—over 2,000 miles from any other land—but it was inhabited by Polynesian 'wayfinders' by 500 AD at the latest and possibly as early as 100 AD. Hawaii's Pacific Ocean neighborhood engulfs a third of our planet and is larger than all our continents combined. It's 995 parts water to 5 parts land, yet almost all of its more than 10,000 islands had been discovered long before European explorers arrived in the region a few centuries ago." (p. 64)

2. *Diversity in Saami terminology for reindeer and snow,* Dr. Ole Henrik Magga. www.arcticlanguages.com/papers/magga_reindeer_and_snow.pdf.

> *The Sami Language,* Department of Scandinavian Studies, The University of Wisconsin-Madison, retrieved 4/18/2011. http://scandinavian.wisc.edu.
>
> ACIA 2005, "Arctic Climate Impact Assessment," Cambridge University Press, p. 973, "The Sami recognize about 300 different quali-

ties of snow and winter pasture, each defined by a separate word in their language."

Chapter 1: Dawn Begins in the Bones

1. Risa Kaparo, lyrics from the poem "Querencia" (song version) on the album *Awaken* (Las Vegas, Nevada: Portal Arts, 2010), www.portalarts. com.

2. Vanda Scaravelli, *Awakening the Spine: The Stress-Free New Yoga That Works with the Body to Restore Health, Vitality and Energy* (San Francisco: HarperOne, 1991), second edition.

3. Alfred Korzybski coined the expression "The map is not the territory" in "A Non-Aristotelian System and its Necessity for Rigour in Mathematics and Physics," a paper presented before the American Mathematical Society at the New Orleans, Louisiana, meeting of the American Association for the Advancement of Science, December 28, 1931. Reprinted in *Science and Sanity,* 1933, pp. 747–61.

4. Bohm lists three kinds of incoherence in our thought:

   1) Thought denies that it is participative;

   2) Thought stops tracking reality and just goes like a program;

   3) Thought establishes its own standard of reference for fixing problems, problems which it contributed to creating in the first place.

5. A term coined my friend, author Steve Bhaerman, coauthor with Bruce Lipton of: *Spontaneous Evolution: Our Positive Future and a Way to Get There from Here* (Carlsbad, California: Hay House, 2003). I appreciate this term, as it describes a self-sustaining, nondual process representing a different paradigm than self-help.

6. Jacques Lusseyran, *And There Was Light* (Sandpoint, Idaho: Morning Light Press, 1987), pp. 26–27.

7. Samuel Bois, *The Art of Awareness,* on the abstracting process (Dubuque, Iowa: W.C. Brown Co., 1966).

Chapter 2: Fundamental Principles of Somatic Learning: The Science and Practice of Awakening Somatic Intelligence

1. Risa Kaparo, from the poem-song "Veils of Sleep," on the album/CD *Awaken* (Las Vegas, Nevada: Portal Arts, 2010), www.portalarts.com.

2. Krishnamurti, from "Authentic Report of Sixteen Talks given in 1945 and 1946" (Whitefish, MT: Kessinger Publishing LLC, 2004), p. 85.

3. Donald O. Hebb, *The Organization of Behavior: A Neuropsychological Theory* (Sussex: Psychology Press, 2002).

4. Daniel J. Siegel, MD, "An Interpersonal Neurobiology Approach to Psychotherapy: Awareness, Mirror Neurons, and Neural Plasticity in the Development of Well-Being," *Psychiatric Annals,* Vol. 36, No. 4 (April 2006).

5. Drs. Rick Hanson and Richard Mendius, from *Meditations to Change Your Brain* audio book (Louisville, CO: Sounds True, 2009). Excerpt from Track 5, 10:20–12:20.

6. Ibid.

7. Ibid.

8. Matthew Sanford, *Waking: A Memoir of Trauma and Transcendence* (Emmaus, PA: Rodale Books, 2008), p. 197.

9. Louise Steinman, *The Knowing Body,* "Proprioception" (Berkeley, California: North Atlantic Books, 1995), second edition, p. 27.

10. Matthew Sanford, *Waking: A Memoir of Trauma and Transcendence,* p. 189.

11. Bruce Lipton, *The Biology of Belief: Unleashing the Power of Consciousness, Matter, and Miracles* (Santa Rosa, California: Mountain of Love/Elite Books, 2005).

12. Daniel J. Siegel, MD, *The Mindful Brain* (New York: W.W. Norton & Company, 2007), pp. 159–62.

13. In *The New Quotable Einstein* (2005), editor Alice Calaprice suggests that two quotes attributed to Einstein that she could not find sources for—"The significant problems we face cannot be solved at the same level of thinking we were at when we created them" and "The world we have created

today as a result of our thinking thus far has problems which cannot be solved by thinking the way we thought when we created them"—may both be paraphrases of the 1946 quote "A new type of thinking is essential if mankind is to survive and move toward higher levels." From "Atomic Education Urged by Einstein," *The New York Times* (May 25,1946), and later quoted in the article "The Real Problem is in the Hearts of Man" by Michael Amrine, *The New York Times Magazine* (June 23, 1946).

14. James and Nora Oschman, "An Expanded View of the Living Matrix," *Massage Therapy Journal,* Vol. 34, No. 3 (Summer 1995).

15. Thomas Hanna, *The Body of Life* (New York: Alfred A. Knopf, 1979), p. 198.

Chapter 3: Engaging the Natural Wisdom of Embodied Mindfulness

1. Deepak Chopra, "Quantum Healing," *Yoga Journal,* No. 87 (July 1989). Published by Active Interest Media, Inc.

2. Francisco J. Varela, Humberto R. Maturana, and R. Uribe (1974), "Autopoiesis: The Organization of Living Systems, Its Characterization and a Model," *Biosystems,* Vol. 5, pp. 187–96. One of the original papers on the concept of autopoiesis.

3. J.L. Oschman (1983), "Structure and properties of ground substances," *American Zoologist 24*(1), pp. 199–215.

4. Joy Brugh, *Joy's Way* (New York: J.P. Tarcher, Inc., 1977).

5. David Bohm, *Wholeness and the Implicate Order* (Great Britain: Routledge, 1980).

6. Peter Levine, PhD, *Waking the Tiger: Healing Trauma* (Berkeley, California: North Atlantic Books, 1997).

7. Thomas Hanna, *The Body of Life* (New York: Alfred A. Knopf, 1979).

8. "Therefore entropy is a complete state of chaos where electromagnetic radiation and energy still exist but are so dispersed as to be effectively nonexistent at a singular point. Eventually (billions and billions of years hence), all suns will have burned out … all planetary motion will have ceased … and all knowledge will have been lost. Thus, the antonym for entropy could be (and often is) stated as 'organized information'. But, I have a

2005). Originally titled *Spiritual Nutrition and the Rainbow Diet,* published by Cassandra Press, 1986).

4. Michael Winn, from the Foreword to *Bone Marrow Nei Kung,* by Mantak Chia (Huntington, New York: Healing Tao Books, 1989).

5. David Bohm, *Wholeness and the Implicate Order.*

6. Posted on www.drweil.com/ "Spirit & Inspiration."

Chapter 7: Bedtime Practices

1. Rumi quote excerpted from "The Dream That Must Be Interpreted," from *The Essential Rumi,* translations by Coleman Barks with John Moyne (New York: HarperOne, 1995).

2. Often we think that we feel more comfortable on soft furniture that conforms to us. Unfortunately, because it doesn't provide the firmness that demands us to find support, we can become more rigid in our tensional patterns. This is most important at night, because having firm support is never as critical as when we are going to sleep. The firmness of the surface provides the resistance that allows us to become as fluid as we are.

3. You can download or purchase a CD or DVD from our website www.awakeningsomaticintelligence.com, where you will also find other useful information, resources, and programs to support your evolving practice.

4. Professor James Oschman is the author of two ground-breaking books, *Energy Medicine: The Scientific Basis* and *Energy Medicine in Therapeutics and Human Performance.* His writing gives even the most skeptical academic scientists a theoretical basis for exploring the physiology and biophysics of energy medicines.

5. Rumi quote from *The Essential Rumi,* translations by Coleman Barks with John Moyne (New York: HarperOne, 1995).

6. Risa Kaparo, from the poem "Awake," in the book *Embrace* (Oakland: Scarlet Tanager Books, 2002).

7. A note on sleeping positions: Generally the safest way to sleep is on your side, with the back slightly curved in a gentle fetal position with the knees and elbows bent. I recommend placing a long pillow (or two smaller

pillows) between your knees and your elbows to avoid compressing the hips or shoulders. Be sure to find a pillow that supports the neck and head—so that the line of the spine remains parallel to your mattress all the way through the head. This requires the support of a good mattress and a pillow of the right size, shape, and texture. You can have yourself measured at a back-support store for a pillow, but generally I find most people do well with a travel-size Tempurpedic® (or similar) pillow, which is easy to adjust as you change positions and to carry with you wherever you go.

8. James and Nora Oschman are directors of Nature's Own Research Association in Dover, New Hampshire. A list of their books and articles can be obtained by writing to P.O. Box 5101, Dover, NH 03820. Telephone 603–742–3789.

9. Werner Heisenberg, as quoted in Fritjof Capra, *The Turning Point: Science, Society, and the Rising Culture* (New York: Random House Digital, Inc., 1983).

Chapter 8: Morning Practices

1. Rumi quote excerpted from the poem "Spring Giddiness" in *The Essential Rumi,* translations by Coleman Barks with John Moyne (New York: HarperOne, 1995).

2. Excerpts from pages 202–204 of *The Poetics of Reverie* by Gaston Bachelard (Ypsilanti, Michigan: Beacon Press, 1971).

Chapter 9: Anytime Anywhere Practices: Standing

1. Risa Kaparo, from the poem "Living On Island" in the book *Embrace* (Oakland: Scarlet Tanager Books, 2002).

2. The term "synesthesia" is generally used in two ways: one to describe a pathological state in which the nervous system crosses senses. The other is used more metaphorically, in poetry for instance, to describe the crossing of metaphors between different senses, like "the taste of green." In the context of Somatic Learning I use the term to speak of the tendency to use a more dominant form of perception to replace a less developed form, even when it doesn't have the same attributes or capacity, such as in the example above.

Chapter 10: Anytime Anywhere Practices: Walking

1. Risa Kaparo, from the poem-song "Water," from the CD *Grateful,* available at www.portalarts.com.

2. Franz Kafka, from "Senses," in *Parables & Paradoxes* (New York: Schocken Books, 1958).

3. To read more on the method of Ideokinesis, I recommend: Lulu E. Sweigard, *Human Movement Potential: Its Ideokinetic Facilitation* (New York: Harper and Row Publishers, Inc., 1974).

4. For more information on forefoot running, see the articles of Rick Williams.

5. Risa Kaparo, from the poem "Overtones" in the book *Embrace* (Oakland: Scarlet Tanager Books, 2002).

6. Adrienne Rich, excerpt from "Transcendental Étude," from *The Dream of a Common Language* (New York: W.W. Norton, 1978), p. 76.

Chapter 11: Anytime Anywhere Practices: Sitting

1. Risa Kaparo, from the poem "The Invocation," published in theartofawakening.com online poetry journal, 2003.

2. Padmasambhava, *Natural Liberation,* translated by B. Alan Wallace (Somerville, Massachusetts: Wisdom Publications, 1998), pp. 105–109.

3. I deepen the experiment in dialogue in an article on "Integrating Multiple Modes of Intelligence." Check www.awakeningsomaticintelligence.com for continuing exploration into these areas.

4. A non-mechanical thought process whereby relevant meaning elevates spontaneously into consciousness following the flow of meaning. This describes the process of insight.

5. See Risa Kaparo, "Somatic Learning Writing Experiments" (I have used "SomaLogics" for the Somatic Learning[sm] dialogue and writing practices) in *E Prime III, An Anthology,* edited by D. Bourland (Concord, CA: International Society of General Semantics, 1997), pp. 289–300.

Chapter 12: Changing Planes/Changing Paradigms

1. Risa Kaparo, from the poem-song "Exequy" on the album/CD *Awaken*. Available at www.portalarts.com.

Chapter 13: Deepening the Dialogue

1. Risa Kaparo, from the poem-song "Everyone I Touch," from the CD/album *Awaken*. Available at www.portalarts.com.

2. Lao Tsu, as quoted in Ruthie Rosauer, *Singing Meditation: Together in Sound and Silence,* Unitarian Universalist Association of Congregations, November 2010.

3. Peter Levine, *Waking the Tiger: Healing Trauma* (Berkeley, California: North Atlantic Books, 1997).

4. Risa Kaparo, phrase from the poem "Querencia" (song version) on the album *Awaken* (Las Vegas, Nevada: Portal Arts, 2010), www.portalarts. com.

5. A recent study showed that "tactile kinesthetic stimulation" (a scientific term for touch) applied for five minutes a day helped premature babies gain an average of 47 percent more weight on the same formula than other babies did. *Journal of Perinatology* 29 (2009), pp. 352–357. Nature Publishing Group.

6. From *Songs of Kabir,* translated by Rabindranath Tagore (Samuel Weiser, Inc., 1977).

Acknowledgements II

It brings me great joy to end this book with a deep bow to all the visionaries who have graced my path. As they are too many to mention here by name, I will limit this list to those whom I have had the great privilege of working with personally, and to explore some of their work in the context of its lineage, in order to give some sense of the varied disciplines—the many rivers that converged into the great sea of meaning in which we will swim together.

A Deep Bow:

To the teachers of Nondual Wisdom and Advaita, especially to my friends Douglas Harding, Isaac Shapiro, Meike Schütt, and Peter Fenner, and to their teachers, Hariwansh Lal Poonja (Papaji), Sai Baba, Ramana Maharshi, and Sri Nisargadatta Maharaj. I am also grateful for my dialogues with Franklin Merrell-Wolff and Bernadette Roberts.

To the visionaries in energy medicine and biology: Bruce Lipton, Karl Maret, MD, Joie Jones, MD, Larry Dossey, MD, Andrew Frankel, MD. Dorian Liebman, PhD, Valerie Hunt, MD, and most especially Nora and James Oschman, PhD, whose ground-breaking scientific papers have inspired and empowered my teaching for the last thirty years.

In the area of birthing, bonding, and early childhood development, I bow to Frederick Leboyer, MD, Michael Odent, MD, Willam Emerson, PhD, Thomas Verny, PhD, Joseph Chilton Pearce, PhD, Jean Liedloff, PhD, James Prescott, PhD, and the attachment theorists.

To the somatic and trauma therapists: Drs. Peter Levine, Ilana Rubenfeld, Francine Shapiro, Robert Williams, Pat Ogden, and especially to the seminal work of Judith Herman, MD.

To the archetypal psychologists: June Singer, PhD, Marion Woodman, PhD, and James Hillman, PhD; and in human potential and mythology: Jean Houston, PhD, Huston Smith, PhD, Joseph Campbell, Angeles

Arrien, Mathew Fox, Michael Mead, Robert Bly, Clarissa Pinkola-Estes, and Martin Shaw. To other therapists and educators with whom I trained: Virginia Satir, PhD, Mel Sudh, PhD, Jack Zimmerman, PhD, Gerry Greenwald, PhD, Edith Sullwald, PhD; and to my mentors in Expressive Arts Therapy, especially Drs. Natalie and Carl Rogers, and in couples work, Drs. David Schnarch and Ruth Morehouse.

To the learning theorist David Boulton, exploring the micro-time dynamics of learning; and in the subject of multi-intelligences, a deep bow to Howard Gardner, PhD, and Daniel Goleman, PhD.

To the interpersonal neurobiologists and neuro-psychologists: especially Daniel Siegal, MD, Rick Hanson, PhD, Richard Mendius, MD, and Stephen Borges, PhD.

To all my teachers of bodywork, cranial-sacral, fascial, visceral, and nerve manipulation, functional integration, structural integration, Jin Shin Jyutsu, Bioenergetics, and Neuro-muscular Re-education, especially to the seminal works of Drs. Moshe Feldenkrais, Ida Rolf, John Upledger, Jean-Pierre Barral, and Thomas Hanna.

To all my teachers of Taoist practices, Tai Chi, Chi Gung, and Aikido: Min Ouyang Si Mu, Judith Weaver, Richard Moon, Mantak Chia, and Share K Lew. To Chaman Lal Kapur, his family, and friends for the opportunity to practice yoga at his ashram in Hoshiarpur, India.

To my teachers of voice and sound healing, including Pandit Pran Nath, Jill Purce, Lisa Rafel, Joshua Leeds, Tito La Rosa, Dolly Kanekuni, Trevor Mitchell, Barbara Juniper, Hilary Reed, Silvia Nakkach, Rhiannon, Heather Houston, Billie Thompson PhD, and her teacher, the father of psycho-acoustics, Alfred A. Tomatis.

To all my mentors in nutrition, functional medicine, and integrative health and to my dear friends and co-conspirators in all of the above: the other founding members of NCSIMH (the Northern California Society of Integrated Mental Health), Jan Hanson, LAc, Tom Reece, ND, Robert Rowend, MD, Kat Toups, MD, and Dorian Leipman, PhD, Dwight Jennings, DDS, Steven Hoskinson, Darick Nordstrom, DDS, Cathy Van Camp and Mark Kline, MD, Ernie Hubbard, Ed Kellogg, PhD,

Susan and Stephen Ducant, PhD, Judy Lane, NP, Mira Hunter, and Rick Williams.

To my teachers of sensory awareness practitioners Charlotte Selver, Charles Brooks, Gerda Alexander, Elsa Middendorf, and Bonnie Bainbridge Cohen.

In poetics: Coleman Barks, Sharon Olds, Tess Gallagher, Richard Silberg, Robert Haas, Carolyn Forche, Brenda Hillman, Richard Garcia, David Whyte, Floyd Salas, Galway Kinnell, and Robert Bly.

In performance art, music, dance, and drumming: Oscar Aguado (later known as Michael Nebadon), Reinhard Flatischler, Heidrun Hoffmann, Mabiba, David Darling, Puna Dawson, Bill Davenport, Gabriel Roth, Koichi and Hiroko Tamano, Eiko and Koma, Mark Shafarman, Tim Mooney, Deborah Eubanks. To all my teachers of contact improvisation, especially Alan Ptashek. And to my Argentine tango teachers, including Rudolfo Dinzel, Gustavo Naveira, Giselle Anne, Luciana Valle, Dana Frigoli, Pablo Villaraza, Somer Sugit, Eugenia Parilla, Chicho Frumbolli, Juana Sepulveda, Paulo Araujo, Miriam Larici and Leonardo Barrionuevo, Norberto "El Pulpo" Esbrés, Luiza Paez, Celine Ruiz, Damian Rosenthal, Juanpablo Guerri, Javier Maldonado, Pablo Alvarez, Milva Bernardi, Daniel Rodriquez, Facundo Jauregui, Daniel Tuero, YuYu Herrera, Maximo Villalba, Oscar Raul Arce, Andrea Fuchilieri, Felipe Martinez, David Orly-Thompson, Mariana Ancarola, and Pouchulu Humberto "El Puchu."

To the other members of my band, The Offering, and to all those who supported the creation of my poetry and music albums, including Alex Acuna, Sophie Barker, Vinnie Colaiuta, Larry Klein, Iki Levy, Mike Rowe, Cameron Stone, Strunz and Farah, Keithen Carter, Robert Irving III, Gary Platt, David Tickle, David Ricketts, Peter Wood, Jon Smith, Cheryl Wilson, Steve Gibbons, Eric Yoder, Richard Famerree, and most especially a deep bow of gratitude to Steve Pressling.

To all my friends along the way who kindly supported me in this and other projects: Demian McKinley, Carol Yamasaki, Lennie Rose, Karen Barrie, Jack Chapman, Annie Barker, David Zimmer, Dia Chass, Brant

Cortright, PhD, Sheila Krystal, PhD, Anna Baldini, Stephen Prucher and Kathleen Ahearn, Craig Rypstat, Amy, Ray and Susanna Laraignee, Ken Donato, Alessandro Moruzzi, Deborah Menges, Tom Taussig, and Gary Platt.

Permissions

The publishers have generously given permission to use excerpts from the following copyrighted works.

From *The Poetics of Reverie* by Gaston Bachelard, translated by Daniel Russell, Copyright © 1969 by Grossman Publishers, Inc. Orig. Copyright © 1960 by Presses Universitaires de France. Used by permission of Viking Penguin, a division of Penguin Group (USA) Inc.

From *Messages From Water,* Vol. 1, Masaru Emoto. Copyright © 1999. Hado Kyoiku Sha Co., Ltd. Reprinted by permission of Office Masaru Emoto, LLC.

From *And There Was Light: Autobiography of Jacques Lusseyran, Blind Hero of the French Resistance,* Jacques Lusseyran. Copyright ©1998. Morning Light Press. Reprinted by permission of Morning Light Press.

From *Natural Liberation: Padmasambhava's Teachings on the Six Bardos,* Padmasambhava. Translated by B. Alan Wallace. Copyright ©1998. Wisdom Publication. Reprinted by permission of The Permissions Company, Inc. on behalf of Wisdom Publications, www.wisdompubs.org

From *Waking: A Memoir of Trauma and Transcendence,* Matthew Sanford. Copyright © 2008. Rodale Books. Reprinted by permission of Rodale Books.

From review of *The Body Electric* by Robert O. Becker, MD, and Gary Selden, by authors of www.newtreatments.org. Reprinted by permission of Etwald Goes.

From *The Essential Rumi,* Coleman Barks / John Moyne. Copyright © 2004 HarperCollins Publishing. Reprinted by permission of Coleman Barks.

James Oschman (1983), "Structure and Properties of Ground Substances," *American Zoologist* 24(1), pp. 199–215.

Index

as neutral force, 58

partnering with, 58–59

transforming your relationship
to, 57–58, 208–9

turning urgency into, xxvii

Gravity-reference scan

lying down, 136–37, 142, 167

sitting, 256

standing, 210–12

Gravity-surfing

birthing and, 114–15

implications of, 128–29

spinal elongation and, 124–27

H

Habituation, cycle of, 43–44

Hanna, Thomas, 34, 57

Hanson, Rick, 21–22, 59

Happiness, enhancing, 22–23

Healing

capacity for, 96

at a distance, 103–5

multi-generational, 15–16

new perspective on, 46–47

presencing and, 11–14

research on, 99–102, 158–60

from trauma, 329–31

Heart, opening the, 225–27

Hebb, Donald, 20

Heisenberg, Werner, 161

Holomovement, 44, 112, 156

Horizon, calling through
sitting, 261–62

standing, 217–18

I

Ideokinetic movement, 247

Insula, 21–22

Internal resources, reallocating,
135–36

Interoception, 22, 42

J

Joyce, James, 155

K

Kabir, 92, 332

Kafka, Franz, 245

Kegel exercises, 116, 185

Keyboard, playing, 278–80

Kidneys, embracing, 314–15

Kinesthesia, 25

Krishnamurti, J., 20, 71, 74, 135, 207

L

Labyrinthine feedback, 25

Lao Tzu, 323

Learning, cycle of, 43–44

Legs, embracing, 310

Levine, Peter, 56

Life

breath as pulse of, 115

enhancing enjoyment of, 13–14,
22–23

Lipton, Bruce, 28–29, 134–35

Love

practice and, 86–87
transformation of water
molecules by, 76–78
Lucidity, 152–53
Lunges
to ground, 295
to standing, 294
Lusseyran, Jacques, 10, 28
LUV sequence, 186–94
Lymphatic system
components of, 121
flushing, 315–16
sensing, 121–22

M

Maturana, Humberto, 45
Meditation. See also Somatic
Meditations
awareness of awareness, 274–75
driving, 281–82
eating, 275–77
happiness and, 22
keyboard, 279–80
sitting, 179–80
walking, 239, 251
Mendius, Richard, 21–22, 59
Mindfulness, embodied. See also
Presencing
effects of, 21–22
as prayer, 104
wisdom of, 25
Mirror, seeing yourself in, 195–96
Morning practices

benefits of, xxx, 156–57, 165
child's pose, 183–86
elongation series, 166–76
implications of, 194–99
LUV sequence, 186–94
missed, xxx
before rising, 154–58
scorpion tail, 180–83
set-up for, 166
sitting forward bend, 176–79
time for, 165
Mozart, Wolfgang Amadeus, 105
Muscle soreness, 94

N

Nathanson, Donald, 91
Natural breathing, 218–20
Natural walking, 245–46
Neuroplasticity, 20–21, 42
Neutral, finding
sitting, 258–60
standing, 212–16
Nondual awareness, 18–19, 25, 73,
106, 113

O

Oliver, Mary, 87
Oral sphincter, 197
Organs, strengthening, 175–76
Oschman, Nora and James, 33, 45,
148, 158–59, 160–61

Prayer
   directed vs. nondirected, 101–2
   effectiveness of, 99–102
   embodied mindfulness as, 104
Presence, extending, xxvii, 53, 55, 74, 94
Presencing. See also Mindfulness, embodied
   efforting vs., 31–32
   healing power of, 11–14, 99
   meaning of, xxvii, 11, 23, 31
Proprioception
   as anchor, 238
   embodied mindfulness and, 42
   focusing vs., 239
   inputs for, 25
   integrating other modes of perception with, 308–9
   meaning of, 25, 26
   unlimitedness of, 101
   visualization vs., 101
Proprioceptive illumination, 28, 34, 35, 43
Prostate gland, 174
Psoas, 312–13

R
Regeneration, 103–4
Ribs
   embracing, 314
   releasing, 170–73
Rich, Adrienne, 250
Rolf, Ida, 159

Rumi, 35, 72, 83, 111, 133, 154, 215
Running, 247–49

S
Sacrum
   anchoring, 125–26
   as key, 201
Sanford, Matthew, 23, 26–28
Scaravelli, Vanda, 4, 85, 86, 87, 92, 216, 244
Scorpion tail, 180–83, 288–91
Selden, Gary, 103–4
Self-facilitation
   from lying supine, 309–10
   outline of elongations, 323–25
   through touch, 305–7
   using the pelvic position with block (or blanket) elongation, 311–15
Self-mastery, 55, 87, 215
Sexual energy, cultivating, 174–75
Shame, 71–72, 89–91
Shape-shifting practice with ball, 145–53
Siegel, Daniel J., 21, 32
Sitting
   awareness of awareness meditation, 274–75
   calling through the horizon, 261–62
   chair, 254–55
   in a chair from standing, 295, 296

at a computer, 278–80

cross-legged, 256–57

finding neutral, 258–60

forward bend, 176–79

meditation, 179–80

pour forward, 265–69, 324

quick spinal release, 269–73

spinal elongation, 263–65

spiral from lying to, 286–87

spiral to lying from, 287–88

Sivander, Gitta, 54

Skull, base of

anchoring, 126, 319

as bowl-shaped diaphragm, 122–23

Slow-motion walking, 240–41

Snake breathing, 127–28

Soft tissue memory, 160–61

Soma-significating, 46

Somatic intelligence

attributes of, 31, 43

awakening of, 13, 28, 30, 34

benefits of developing, xxvi, xxvii, 4, 18, 33

maturation of, 56

non-local healing and, 103–5

pervasiveness of, 55

potential of, 100

Somatic Learning. See also Somatic Learning experiences

beliefs and, 30–31

benefits of, 4, 12, 14, 18–19, 57–58, 88–89

embodiment and, 23

healing and, 46–47

implications of, 52–53

inquiry and, 53

intention of, 33, 63–65

motivations for interest in, 3–4

session design for, 53

touch in, 325

Somatic Learning experiences

author's, 6–13

Carrie (birthing), 114–15

Charles (knee problems), 283–84

David (spinal cord injury), 298–301

Ellen (becoming lightness, ease, and comfort), 209

Joan (dancing without pain), 162

Katrama (creating space and transforming structure), 163

Kay (aging gracefully), 107

Larry (multi-generational healing), 15–16

Lisa (transforming a health crisis), 96–98

Marty (transforming chronic pain), 79–81

Reka (beyond apparent limitation), 235–36

Ron (moving from contraction into pleasure), 130–31

Telephone, talking on, 197

Tenzin, Lama Pema, 103

Thighs, embracing, 312–13

Thoughts, power of, xxxv

Thriving vs. surviving, 20–21

Thubten, Anam, 275

Tidal breath, 117

Time, as neutral force, 58

Tomkins, Silvan, 69, 91

Tonglin, 180

Touch
    facilitating others through,
      325–31
    limited access to, 330
    self-facilitation through, 305–7

Trauma, healing from, 329–31

U

Umbilicus, embracing, 318–19

Uribe, Ricardo, 45

Urinary sphincter, 196

Uttanasana, 176–79

V

Varela, Francisco, 45

Vestibular feedback, 25

Visceral feedback, 25

Visualization, 101, 102

Visual perception, overreliance on,
  26

W

Walking
    with arm wheel, 241–45
    downhill, 246
    ideokinetic movement, 247
    meditation, 239, 251
    natural, 245–46
    slow-motion, 240–41
    uphill, 246

Water molecules, transformation of,
  76–78

Weight-shifting, 212–16

Weil, Andrew, 128

Weiss, Paul, 159

Whyte, David, 74

Winn, Michael, 120

Women, health concerns of, 173–74

Wounding
    regeneration and, 103–4, 158–60
    research on, 99–102

Wren, Maurice, xxxiii

Writing, 277–78

Y

Young, J. Z., 158–59, 160–61

Z

Zakili, Katayoon Zand, 54

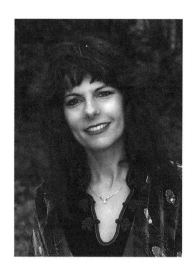

About the Author

A licensed psychotherapist, Risa Kaparo, PhD, is the developer of Somatic Learning, a bodymind approach to self-healing and self-renewal that incorporates psychological, somatic, yogic, and meditative disciplines. She has developed training programs for health professionals and educators, and has taught Somatic Learning at MIT, John F. Kennedy University, the California Institute of Integral Studies, Dalian Medical University in China, and numerous other universities and professional institutions. Dr. Kaparo is a licensed minister and directs Inquiry, a division of The Association for the Integration of the Whole Person, a non-denominational, non-sectarian religious non-profit. Her recently released companion video, *Awakening Somatic Intelligence: The Art and Practice of Embodied Mindfulness,* beautifully demonstrates the transformational practices she teaches in the book and features documentary style interviews with practitioners that convey the life-changing effects of this work. She offers an additional series of CDs and DVDs on Somatic Learning.

Risa Kaparo is also an award-winning poet and songwriter. She is the author of *Embrace* (Scarlet Tanager Press) and two albums of poetry and music, *Awaken* and *Grateful* (Portal Arts), which express her passion for awakening through a spirituality of sensuousness—loving what is. Grand prize winner of the John Lennon Songwriting Contest, Kaparo appears internationally as a poet performance artist and dancer. She maintains a private somatic psychotherapy practice in the San Francisco Bay Area.